TREAD LIGHTLY

FORM, FOOTWEAR, AND THE QUEST
FOR INJURY-FREE RUNNING

Peter Larson and Bill Katovsky

Skyhorse Publishing

Skyhorse Publishing books may be purchased in bulk at special discounts for sales promotion, corporate gifts, fund-raising, or educational purposes. Special editions can also be created to specifications. For details, contact the Special Sales Department, Skyhorse Publishing, 307 West 36th Street, 11th Floor, New York, NY 10018 or info@skyhorsepublishing.com.

Skyhorse® and Skyhorse Publishing® are registered trademarks of Skyhorse Publishing, Inc.®, a Delaware corporation.

Visit our website at www.skyhorsepublishing.com.

Cover photo courtesy of Merrell

This book provides extensive information about running injuries, running footwear, running form, and nutrition. In the process of presenting these topics, we discuss numerous scientific articles, books, and other publications. Any errors in quotation or interpretation are the fault of the authors, and not of the sources.

Information presented in this book does not constitute medical advice. Outcomes resulting from choosing new footwear, altering running form, and making changes to your training can be difficult to predict, and injuries are possible. We recommend consulting with a qualified medical practitioner prior to making any change.

10 9 8 7 6 5 4 3 2 1

Library of Congress Cataloging-in-Publication Data is available on file.
ISBN: 978-1-61608-374-8

Printed in the United States of America

To Erin, Anders, Emma, and Benjamin.
Your understanding, support, and patience
made this book possible.

—PML

Each of us is an experiment of one—observer and subject—making choices, living with them, recording the effects.

—George Sheehan, M.D.

Contents

Preface

When you come to think of it, some few (comparatively) cen-
turies ago there was only one law which appealed to all and
sundry. But its appeal was imperative. Four words will cover
it—"Eat, or be eaten." In those days mankind had to rely on
legs to be in a position to carry out the first part or evade the
latter. So everyone ran and ate; when they failed to run fast or
far enough they met the eater . . . at that time instinct kept the
race perpetually fit.

—ARTHUR NEWTON, *RUNNING*, 1935

Legendary South African ultrarunner Arthur Newton recognized something very important when he wrote the above passage in his 1935
book titled "*Running.*" Decades before Christopher McDougall shook up
many conventional beliefs about running with a bestselling book about
his experience with the Tarahumara Indians of Mexico's Copper Canyon,
Newton realized that humans were natural born runners. Newton was
like many of today's runners—he didn't start running seriously until he
was 38 years old, and the initial experience of going just two miles left
him stiff for several days.

An autodidact when it came to running, Newton loved to experiment
with different training methods and approaches to fueling and hydration,
including making an energy drink from lemonade and salt. He tended
to think a lot about running form, finding that his perfect stride length
was three feet, seven inches, and that his ideal footwear were cheap can-

vas sneakers with crepe-rubber soles that seldom needed replacing. He regularly logged over 500 running miles per month, won the Comrades Marathon several times, and set multiple ultramarathon world records (including at 60 and 100 miles). His 24-hour distance record of 152 miles stood for over two decades.

As the world's best endurance runner at the time, Newton was somewhat of a fitness proselytizer, like an earlier version of Dr. George Sheehan and Jim Fixx, both of whom also became born-again runners in early middle age. The South African athlete passionately believed that it was entirely possible for anyone who put in the necessary time and effort to become a runner. Yet Newton was a realist who acknowledged that the average man of his day was in a fairly poor physical state: "the physique of the ordinary individual is not cut out for, nor reasonably capable of, sudden enormous exertions such as are entailed by a twenty-six mile race, owing to the adverse conditions brought about by modern civilization."

Few people nowadays would disagree with Newton's observation. *Homo sapiens* is a running species, but modern society for the most part has shunned running or exercise with any level of regularity. And those of us who do decide to take up running are often saddled with chronic or recurring injuries, and are left wondering why.

Could many of our running-injury woes be tied directly to unhealthy aspects of a modern lifestyle? Most of us simply don't live like our ancestors; nor do we tend to use our body in the manner that drove its evolution to its current state. Instead of hunting and gathering and being active for a good portion of the day, we tend to be sedentary and eat heavily processed and sugary foods rather than fresh meats, fruits, and vegetables. Even serious runners often find that much of their day is spent slouched in an office chair in front of a computer, all the while wearing shoes that can impact their anatomy and biomechanics. When the runner finally makes it out the door for a workout, it's usually on unyielding, unvarying man-made surfaces instead of sand, dirt, and irregular rocky terrain. The list could go on and on.

Our goal in writing *Tread Lightly* was not to provide an exhaustive review of how modern life negatively affects one's health and running, but rather to examine three specific changes that are of particular importance and relevance: footwear, form, and food.

We start at the beginning and discuss how man developed his unique running prowess through evolution via natural selection. From there we move on to a discussion why we *should* run and why we tend to get hurt while doing so. We then focus on footwear history and how shoes and gait play a significant role in both causing and correcting the ills of the modern runner. Nutrition is examined in this context. By weaving together information pulled from experts, coaches, doctors, and scientists, we hope to make the strong and persuasive argument that running should be enjoyable, and not a source of discomfort, pain, or serial misery. Once you're armed with the knowledge obtained from this book, it's our hope that you will be able to look at running in a whole new light.

—Peter Larson and Bill Katovsky
April 2012

Introduction

Out on the roads there is fitness and self-discovery and the persons we were destined to be.

—George Sheehan, M.D.

Pete's Story

How does a college professor in the hard sciences develop an obsession with running shoes? It's an interesting question and one that I often ask myself when gearing up for a run and choosing from among the over fifty pairs of colorful shoes that comprise my collection. Professors are supposed to wear sensible shoes and tweed jackets with elbow patches, not tech gear and flashy racing flats with bright orange flames on the sides. I have a problem, and I openly admit it—shoes fascinate me, but not for reasons of aesthetics or status. Instead, I'm curious about how footwear is designed and how shoes allow one's body to work. I teach human anatomy and exercise physiology, so the study of form and function is what gets my creative and analytical juices flowing at full speed.

My running shoe infatuation is a relatively new affliction. There was a time when I didn't care much about shoes, or give them much thought. So how did I get to this point, when the arrival of a new pair of shoes at my doorstep via UPS or FedEx is cause for a small internal celebration? Let's start from the beginning.

I am thirty-seven years old, and I've been a runner off and on for much of my life. I played soccer and tennis in high school, both of which involved a healthy dose of both jogging and wind sprints, but at the time

I viewed running more as punishment than pleasure. At that age, we just ran when the coach told us to, and complained about it to each other afterward. I was in excellent shape, and I remember vividly the triumphant moment when I first successfully ran the three-mile test for soccer in under twenty-one minutes—that was the time I needed to make varsity. I nearly vomited from the exertion put into that run, but I think that was the moment I realized the joy and exhilaration that comes with reaching a new running milestone. My shoe of choice back then was a loud-looking pair of André Agassi tennis shoes decked out in neon yellow and black— it's one of the few pairs of shoes from my past that retains a place in my mental memory bank.

As a college student at the University of Richmond, my relationship with running became strained. I put on the typical freshman 15 pounds (and then some), and I essentially stopped running for the better part of four years. In graduate school at Ohio University, I picked the sport back up and had my first encounter with an overuse injury directly caused by a bad pair of shoes. My primary criterion for choosing a shoe was the same as it had been in high school: the shoe that looked best was the one that found its way onto my foot—aesthetics reigned over function. The Adidas shoes that I was wearing at the time were a half-size too large, but they were brightly colored and looked fast, and that's all that really mattered to me. Unfortunately, my legs paid the price, and one day on a run over the hills of Southeast Ohio, I started to feel a burning sensation along the side of my thigh, just above the knee. Eventually it got to the point where the pain was excruciating, particularly on the downhills, and I can vividly remember limping home in agony on more than one run. I determined that I had iliotibial band syndrome (ITBS), which is an inflammation of a band of connective tissue that extends downward from the pelvis, along the outer portion of the thigh, and connects to the tibia just below the knee joint.

I read somewhere that shoes can be the culprit in ITBS, so I ditched the ill-fitting pair and the pain gradually went away. It was like voodoo; remove the shoe—remove the pain, but I didn't really think too much of it at the time (my running shoe infatuation had yet to begin). I kept on running through most of graduate school, often on an indoor track, and never more than two to three miles. I couldn't fathom the idea of going any longer than that.

The end of graduate school commenced yet another period of inactivity and slothfulness in my life. Rather than accept a prestigious postdoctoral research fellowship that I had been awarded at a large university, I opted to take a job as a professor at Saint Anselm College, a small, teaching-oriented college in New Hampshire, where I am still employed today. Teaching has always been my passion, and the location was ideal for me and my wife since it was close to our families and we were expecting our first child.

The stress-inducing combination of a being a new faculty member and the arrival of my first son at the end of my first semester sucked away all of my free time. If I happened to wear a pair of running shoes for the next three and a half years, it wasn't for anything more strenuous than mowing the lawn. Running had been banished from my world.

A few years later a second child arrived on the scene, following my wife's very difficult and stressful pregnancy. With exercise non-existent and the food scraps from both of my kids' plates finding their way onto mine, the extra pounds began to accumulate on my 5'10" frame. And before I knew it, I was about twenty pounds overweight. I think it was probably the heaviest I had ever been in my life. I was disgusted with the fact that I had let myself go so far, and then it happened.

The moment of truth, or rather the wake-up call, was a photograph. It was a simple image that changed my life, and sent me on a journey that would eventually carry me through thousands of miles, eight marathons, and an ultra (and counting), and owning more pairs of running shoes than I care to admit.

The photo was taken in May 2007 at a Saint Anselm College commencement ceremony. That particular commencement had special personal meaning because it was for the graduating class that entered the college as freshmen during my first year as a newly minted member of the faculty. Like any commencement ceremony, the aftermath was filled with hugs, goodbyes to students who felt more like family after struggling together through the previous four years, and lots of pictures. I received one of these photos via email from a student a few days later, and what I saw in that image horrified me.

I'm generally not overly concerned with my appearance, but when it comes to body weight I fight a constant battle. I've never been what I would call obese, but what I saw in that picture was somebody who was downright pudgy. I had, in that photograph, become something that I

had feared for my entire life—a fat man. And I couldn't take my eyes off
of it. I needed to make a change. So I started, once again, to run. Only
this time, as the pounds slowly melted off with each mile run, my physique wasn't the only thing that changed. Rather, my entire outlook toward running changed, and it became something more than just a hobby.
It became an essential, almost all-encompassing part of my life.

Initially I ran just short distances, but my wife and I both decided to
enter a four-mile road race in Bridgton, Maine in the summer of 2007,
and I needed to put in enough miles to be certain I could finish (I had
never run four miles before). The motivation that the looming race provided was incredible, and it reignited a competitive fire in me that seemed
to have been extinguished since high school. I was amazed to find that I
could run three miles without passing out, and my mileage slowly began
to creep upward. But along with the ramp-up in mileage came problems,
I began experiencing some knee and shin pain, so I took the advice of a
colleague at work (an experienced runner) and decided it was time to buy
a proper pair of running shoes. I was wearing a pair of ASICS trail shoes
that I bought, once again, because they looked cool, and suspected that
they might be playing a role in causing my pain. I headed to a local specialty running store, and left with a pair of Nike Air Structure Triax shoes
that was supposedly perfectly suited to how I ran.

So began my real running life. With my fancy new shoes, I ran through
the four-mile race in Maine, and then a few more local 5K's and a 10K.
Each new race seemed to bring a new PR, and the desire for personal
improvement became addictive. I'm both a perfectionist and extremely
self-competitive—I don't really care who finishes in front of or behind
me, but I'm always in a race to the death against myself. I ended my first
racing season by completing the inaugural and ridiculously hilly Manchester City Half-Marathon in 1:41:24—not blazing fast by any means,
but fast enough for me, especially since the race was ten miles longer than
I had ever run just a short six months prior. I was hooked, and there was
no turning back.

I actually wore down the heel of that first pair of Nikes straight
through to the point where I deflated the air chamber on one side, which
caused the heel to go all mushy, like a car with a flat tire (an early con-
firmation that I was a serious heel scuffer). For its replacement, I chose a
stability shoe, because that's what the clerk at the specialty running store

told me I needed, and the thought of hurting myself if I deviated was always lurking in my head. Getting injured was not an option—the sport had become an essential part of my life in far too many ways for me to cope with being sidelined for any length of time.

Things began to change for me on the running shoe front when my race times started to drop in late 2008. I began reading that a lighter shoe could help shave off a few additional seconds from my times by making my running more efficient (less weight at the end of the leg meant less energy expended). I decided to buy a pair of Saucony Fastwitch 2's, a lightweight training shoe that offered some stability; I logged personal records in both the 5K and half-marathon in them. Regardless of whether the shoes or my improved training and conditioning deserved credit for the faster race times, I was happy with my transition into lighter-weight footwear, and I was primed for what was to come.

My running-shoe obsession intensified early in 2009 when I read Christopher McDougall's *Born to Run*, which focused in part on the problems with modern running shoes. *Born to Run* didn't make me want to throw away my shoes; rather what the book did was force me think about my footwear *and* question why exactly I was wearing the shoes that I put on my feet. As an anatomist and evolutionary biologist who did his dissertation research in an animal locomotion lab (though I studied tadpole anatomy and biomechanics of all things!), I was familiar with many of the scientists McDougall cited in *Born to Run*. His discussion of biomechanics and the evolution of running was right up my professional alley. The scientist in me wanted to know more—a lot more.

Born to Run triggered something internal: I felt betrayed by my own unhealthy reliance on cushy running shoes, which were apparently double agents, undermining my body's apparently innate desire to allow my foot to lightly kiss the ground with each stride. Where I should have been springing down the road on my forefeet, I was instead pounding the pavement with my heel on each and every step. I'd never thought about this before, and to be honest, I'd never had much reason to. Unlike McDougall, who was searching for answers about why one of his feet hurt, both of mine felt just fine. In fact, I had been remarkably injury free since those first few weeks as a runner, even though I had been wearing the very style of arch-supporting, pronation-preventing shoe that McDougall was railing against.

I began to wonder—did it really matter what I wore? Was it really all about the shoes? Did the fact that I was a confirmed heel striker make a difference?

Driven by restless curiosity, I had to find answers. I started reading everything I could find about the biomechanics of running and the science behind shoes. I began thinking and writing out loud on a personal blog called *Runblogger*. I began experimenting with different kinds of footwear and different running gaits. I even initiated a research project with some of my undergraduates to film marathon runners in order to analyze their footstrikes. I learned a lot in a short period of time (and I'm still learning every day), and among the things I discovered was that pronation, which is the inward roll of the foot after it contacts the ground, is not necessarily the evil enemy of all runners as we are so often made to believe. I learned that extensive cushioning is not a requirement for comfortable running on a hard surface. I also discovered that one's footwear does in fact change how one runs, but that the implications of these gait changes continue to be the subject of heated debate.

Buttressed with this new scientific wisdom to ignore advice about such things as pronation-control, I bought a pair of ultra-light, ultra-flexible, neutral cushioned (gasp!) Nike Free 3.0's. To my amazement and happiness, running in the Nike Frees was a liberating experience—it felt like I was running in well-cushioned slippers. I ran twenty miles on my third run in them, and though I suffered through some serious muscle soreness in my legs, I survived my own direct assault on the pronation-control paradigm. Stability shoes be damned! I knew that I could never go back to running in the heavy traditional trainers that now felt like bricks strapped to my feet.

Shortly after transitioning into the Nike Frees I purchased a pair of Vibram FiveFingers KSO's, the ultra-minimal foot-gloves made famous by McDougall and "Barefoot" Ted McDonald in *Born to Run*. The Vibrams were in an entirely different league than even the Frees. With no heel, minimal cushion, and little individual pockets for each toe, they were unlike anything I had ever attempted to run in. The biggest difference that I noticed on my first Vibram run was that they almost immediately made me get off my heels (even the Nike Frees, with their ample midsole cushioning, hadn't accomplished that). This was both good and bad. The good was that the shoes were working as advertised, the bad was that I wasn't used to landing on my forefoot and I managed to overdo it. I felt some pain in my right forefoot on landings and had some soreness on the top of my foot for several days afterward. I shelved the VFF's for a few weeks to make sure I didn't seriously aggravate anything.

My second run in the Vibrams was also a case of doing too much too soon—I ran seven miles, and I paid the price. By night, my legs were stiff, but I wasn't hurting. When I woke up the next morning, however, I knew I was in trouble—my calves were screaming, and I could barely walk without pain. Despite my legs begging for some rest, I decided to still go out for my planned long run (yes, I'm quite capable of being both stubborn and stupid), and the soreness trimmed my 17 miler into a 13 mile walk/run nightmare. My calves were on fire and I was hobbling around like I had just finished a marathon. It was at that point that I realized there was something to this minimalist shoe movement. The pain wasn't a bad thing. Changing shoes had changed my gait, and changing my gait had changed how my leg muscles were being worked. My leg muscles were sore because they were weak. They simply needed time to get stronger.

The intial soreness was short-lived, and I slowly built up my mileage in my FiveFingers, careful to only run in them once a week or so. It was hard to limit myself, simply because running in the shoes was so much fun. I felt like a kid who was sticking his tongue out at the shoe gods, and every mile that I logged in Vibrams was a personal attack on the status quo. I had been told I needed stability, but here I was wearing what amounted to a foot-glove, and short of occasional bouts of delayed onset muscle soreness in my calves, I wasn't getting hurt. I was, however, getting stronger, and my Vibram journey eventually took me on runs as long as fifteen miles.

On *Runblogger*, I wrote about my ongoing experiment with minimalist shoes and running form, and through my involvement with the online running community I began to meet kindred souls. Other runners were experimenting as well, and our numbers were growing. Some were overcoming nagging injuries by trying something different, yet others were experiencing various problems with the transition to a more natural running style. We were all learning in the process.

My initial curiosity with minimalist, barefoot-style running shoes eventually led me to start reviewing them in depth. My full-fledged shoe obsession was now underway. A seemingly never-ending stream of shoes, both self-purchased and media samples sent by footwear manufacturers, began to make their way into our house. It has become a joke for my wife and kids to shout at the UPS or FedEx truck to "*keep going, keep going!*" as it approaches our driveway. When the truck does stop, my initial reaction is to act excited (which I am). My wife pretends to get angry, but I know she's only pretending (I think). She's also a runner, but sadly does not share my footwear fetish.

This is what passes for fun in the Larson household these days. As a full-fledged and proud-to-be shoe addict, when I am not busy preparing for lectures, grading exams, changing diapers, or shuttling my older kids to various extracurricular activities, I find myself weighing shoes on a postage scale, measuring heel and forefoot heights with calipers, and photographing the shoes on our dining room table. All of this is done in the name of running shoe science, while my poor wife simply shakes her head, wondering how she got stuck married to this lunatic.

So, in the course of nearly five years, I've gone from becoming an overweight, largely sedentary slug who couldn't care less about running, let alone running shoes, to being a relatively fit runner with a 3:15 Boston-qualifying time for the marathon. In the process of getting healthy, I've developed a full-blown obsession with the design, functionality and the nitty-gritty science of running footwear. Runners often say that the sport can change your life, and in my case this couldn't be truer. Running has brought me to the point where I am right now, writing this book with my coauthor Bill Katovsky, hoping to share some of the knowledge (and mistakes) we have learned during this exciting journey of self-discovery.

Now it's his turn to describe his own journey as a runner. Just like with my own, it had its share of ups and downs. There was even at extended period, much longer than mine in fact, when he didn't run at all. Of the two of us, I'm more the analytical and competitive one. I wear a GPS-watch, log every run, and pore over pacing and mileage. I shoot for personal records and run myself into the ground in every race. I read esoteric scientific papers on running form and footwear and find them to be fascinating springboards for personal experimentation. Bill, on the other hand, despite being a two-time Hawaii Ironman finisher and founder of *Tri-Athlete* magazine, is a self-described running romanticist—he never runs with a watch, seldom competes in races anymore, loves running alone on hilly trails, and savors every moment when his shoe bottoms are lightly kissing the ground and his thoughts are traveling far, far away. Yet, despite our differences, we are both runners interested in the changing landscape of our sport.

❧

Bill's Story

Since I'm fifteen years older than Pete, as he was learning to stand up and walk, I was sucking wind during high school soccer practice sprints, running from one end of the field to the other. Later, at the University of Michigan, the most I ever ran was one mile on the gym's rickety indoor wooden track—eight laps to a mile—before hitting the weight room. I hated running. A guy on my dorm floor ran seven miles every morning, even in the snow and rain. I never asked him why. I just assumed that his daily running ritual made him weirder than he already was. His sink-washed white tube socks were always drying on the radiator in his room.

The sport I loved was long-distance cycling. The summer before my senior year, I biked solo across the United States. After I graduated from college and headed out west again, this time to take a seasonal job as firefighter in Montana, the idea of running began to present intriguing possibilities. I wanted to become a smokejumper, the airborne elite of wild lands firefighting, but part of the qualifying process was the ability to run ten miles. I parked that number deep inside my brain and in early fall, while I was hanging out in Yosemite for a month, I became a runner. Because I was in terrific hiking shape, I got up to two, then three, and finally five miles without much difficulty. Running turned into something fun. I wore Tretorn tennis sneakers.

Running then followed me back East to Washington, D.C., where I spent a year as a political researcher at the Brookings Institute. After work and on weekends, I would run along the Potomac, either past the Watergate Hotel complex and Jefferson Memorial or along the canal towpath that started in Georgetown. My longest runs had now edged up to eight miles. I never ran with a watch, and I was still doing a lot of biking. Although this was 1980 and I wasn't yet familiar with concepts like cross-training or the existence of some newfangled endurance race called the Hawaii Ironman triathlon, the combination of cycling and running seemed to ward off any knee or leg injuries.

It was then out West, once more, not to become a firefighter in Montana, since my application to the U.S. Forest Service had been rejected, but to Berkeley, after having been accepted into the political science doctoral program. Bogged down with the pressure of taking classes and studying, I only ran twice a week, usually for two miles on the university track or along the dirt fire road and hiking trail in Strawberry Canyon that snaked upward from the campus into the Berkeley Hills.

These two running venues couldn't have been more different in terms of terrain and setting. The steep, narrow canyon was lined with eucalyptus and oak trees; running there always felt secluded, private, peaceful. But on the quarter-mile track at Edwards Stadium, I had company with other runners and hurdlers. I was a slave to the sweeping second hand of my wristwatch. My interest was in speed, not solitude. I'd run the first mile in about seven minutes and the second one between 6:15 and 6:30. Afterwards, I would lay sprawled on the infield grass, gulping down oxygen as if from a Krazy Straw.

One late afternoon at the track, there was an all-comers meet. Anyone could race! So I chose to compete in the 440. There were about a dozen of us. I seeded myself in the rear. A volunteer track coach was the timer. When he blew his whistle, I tentatively followed in the caboose, unsure how to pace myself. But when you've run countless laps on the same track, you begin to know its familiar curves as intimately as you would any lover. By the second turn, I was mid-pack, and holding steady. Third turn, the same. Right before the homestretch, I mentally prepared myself for the inevitable: going all out. Those final hundred or so yards, I smoked the field and finished first in 60 seconds flat. Proud of my unexpected triumph, I walked over to the track coach who was also the meet organizer. He was in his early sixties and wore a polyester tracksuit.

After regaining my breath, I asked him, "So what do you think? Do I have any promise as a runner?"

He glared at me as if I had just told him that his fly was open. "You run all wrong. You ran on your heels the entire time."

I was about to ask him why that was such a bad thing or better yet, what was the *right* way to run a short race like the 440. But I kept silent and walked away. It was the last time I ran on Edwards Track. My running was my own personal affair, ruled not by white-striped corridors on an oval track or the judgmental scorn of others.

The following year, I impulsively entered my first running race—a 13.1-mile hilly affair that started in Berkeley. I was running between ten and fifteen miles a week in tennis sneakers. I hadn't trained specifically for this race. Earlier that week, I had come across a flyer for the Berkeley-to-Moraga half-marathon in a bookstore on Telegraph Avenue. I was curious about running that far. The farthest I had ever run was ten miles in a single stretch and that had been back in D.C. Since I seldom ran with a watch, I didn't care a whit about a predicted time, nor did I even know what to shoot for.

When I showed up on that cold fall morning near the driveway entrance to the grand-looking Claremont Hotel, there were about two hundred runners already gathered on a side street, many hopping about in order to stay warm. Almost everyone seemed to know one another. I noticed several guys wearing red or blue running tights. I had never seen that before. I thought runners only wore shorts.

Same racing script as before: I seeded myself in the back and waited for the half-marathon to begin. The first 4.5 miles went straight uphill, first along a steep section of Ashby Avenue and then over to the switch-backing Tunnel Road, where all the homes would later go up in smoke in the devastating 1991 Oakland fire. I started out too fast and struggled in oxygen debt, but I edged back, recovered my wind, and paced myself on the gradual climb. I must have been in the top half of the field at the 1,200-foot summit, feeling cocky and smug at my success; but on the subsequent two-mile flat section, runner after runner zipped right past me. My legs felt leaden and unresponsive.

The course descended into a heavily forested canyon for several miles. Near the eight- or nine-mile mark, I asked a female runner who had pulled alongside me, "How are you feeling? Tired?" My legs had the consistency of concrete.

"No," she replied. "I feel fine."

"I'm curious, but can you tell me how much training you do?"

"About thirty or forty miles a week," she replied, before peeling away. There was no way I could keep up with her.

Running is a numbers game, I thought. You need to put in the training mileage to do well in a race. I fought through the remaining miles, finishing in a mental and physical fog. My time was 1:45, or just over eight minutes per mile. Someone handed me a small, yellow fabric finisher's patch. I never checked the final standings to see where I placed, though there was a posting of just the top ten times—they were all in the seventy-minute range. The following day, I came down with the flu and spent the next seventy-two hours shaking and shivering in bed because I had overstressed my immune system. My body paid the penalty for being undertrained.

Yes, training. Pretty much a foreign concept to someone who simply liked running for its intrinsic enjoyment and health benefits. But training was what I began to do, and *needed* to do, after taking some time off from grad school in order to get in shape for the 1982 Hawaii Ironman. My run mileage increased to about twenty to twenty-five miles a week. I even bought genuine running shoes from a small specialty store tucked on a side street in downtown Oakland by Lake Merritt. Walking into the cluttered space with running shoe boxes stuffed ceiling high, I was overwhelmed by the smell of factory-fresh rubber and variety of brands. I left with a box of Nike Pegasus shoes under my arm and stayed with this model for years to follow.

These shoes got me through 500 miles of training, and more importantly, the third segment of the Ironman—the marathon—though my body almost didn't because of a severely strained calf muscle that happened moments after the start of the 2.4-mile ocean swim. Biking for 112 miles in the hot, windy conditions further aggravated the calf injury. For weeks leading up to the race, I had made a private sworn-to-the-athletic-gods promise not to walk any of the marathon. That oath was broken before I left the town of Kona and made it to the Queen K lava desert highway. *Only* twenty miles remained in the run. Hobbling, shuffling, walking, running when I could bear the pain, I somehow willed myself not to quit. With an adrenaline rush spurring me toward the end, I ran hard those last few miles and finished two hours before the mandatory midnight deadline. It was one of the greatest athletic triumphs in my life. Several months later, I launched a new magazine for the young sport. I named it *Tri-Athlete*.

Tri-Athlete quickly became successful and I sold it after three years. Throughout this period, I kept in shape by biking and running several hours a week. I was fortunate to have a great motivational workout asset: my dog named Rockee, a wild-at-heart golden retriever who loved to run.

We were joined at the hip for fourteen years and 7,000 miles of running together. Rockee was a seventy-pound bundle of crazy canine affection. He never once complained if we ran too far or were going too slowly. I never heard him go on and on about an injury, like so many runners do. He never bellyached if the weather was too hot or too cold. Or about setting a PR in his next race. He just loved to run. His limitless energy and unflagging enthusiasm were inspiring to behold. Each time I put on my Pegasus shoes, running shorts, and bandana, he'd go into an uncontrollable state of insane delight and expectation, bouncing, twisting and corkscrewing in midair like a demented acrobat.

Rockee helped me get in shape for my second Hawaii Ironman—eleven years after my first race. I was now living in Boulder where a sports publisher had hired me to relaunch a new triathlon magazine. (During the previous seven years, I had been far removed from the triathlon scene and had stayed in the Bay Area where I ran two magazines, one on literature and the arts, and the other a lifestyle glossy for San Francisco, cheekily named *Frisko*.)

After spending a year in Boulder, I returned to the Bay Area. Rockee and I continued our collaborative running along narrow trails and dusty fire roads in Marin County. Then old age and arthritis finally caught up with him. Our two-hour runs dwindled to short, slow-paced walks.

It was a horrible, horrible day when he died in my arms at the vet due to rapid blood loss resulting from a ruptured spleen. I cried for a week. Maybe two weeks. A dark, hollow emptiness spread inside me and just kept increasing. An unfathomable sadness, I realized, would be my new companion. I lost almost all interest in running. Occasionally, I would go on a half-hour or hour run, but it never seemed the same without Rockee right by my side. Memories are a man's best friend.

And thus began my steady fitness decline in my early 40s, a physical deterioration emotionally amplified by watching my father slowly succumb to Alzheimer's, then fighting my own battle with depression. I also came down with dermatitis and edema in both legs that were most likely caused by an unwise addiction to Advil (averaging thirty or forty pills a day) to help me relax and sleep. I kept busy writing and editing books on the media and politics, but these melancholic and miserable years grinded on like this, a continuing downward spiral that was also marked by never breaking a sweat or going for a run. When I hit fifty, the reality of how far

I had bottomed out in terms of fitness was too powerful to ignore. It was time for a lifestyle change.

I had tried once before to reverse the physical decline, but it turned out to be a false and premature attempt to regain control over what had happened to my slack body. Somewhere into the sixth or seventh year of my Lost Fitness Decade, I bought a pair of New Balance all-terrain running shoes. Since I had been away from running for so long, I thought that my weakened feet and ankles would need the extra support that a honking-big, thick-tread, large-heel shoe could hopefully deliver. The product literature for the NB 101's promised a "lightweight compression molded EVA midsole for cushioning and flexibility," and an "aggressive solid rubber lugged outsole" that could pound nails into sheetrock if I happened to misplace a hammer, not that I did any carpentry. I thought that a new pair of running shoes would provide the incentive to start running again. But who was I kidding? For several years, the shoes sat unused in their box in a closet, the pitiful reminder of an ill-conceived, over-the-phone purchase from LL Bean.

When I finally decided to start running again, I certainly didn't feel like a runner, nor did I deserve to be considered one, not on that first day when I could barely trot up the 75-yard driveway in a pair of heavy leather and rubber-soled clogs. When I reached the mailbox, I was breathing hard, legs unsteady and shaking. I followed this same "workout" routine for several days, still wearing the clogs. I then progressed to super-slow jogging for about two hundred yards along the dead end street to a splintering wooden guardrail that became my finish line. The road had a gradual incline. This meager distance represented my absolute physical limit. My quads and calves ached. Every breath was forced and labored. The exertion drained me. I would walk home.

I was amazed by how strange running had become. I was aware of every plodding foot strike. My body's herky-jerky awkwardness would have been laughable—if only it were happening to someone else. A disconnect existed between my upper and lower body, as if I were put together from mismatched parts and faulty electrical wiring.

I continued with the jogging-and-walking routine for about a month. I got up to one mile. Sometimes a clog would slip off if I was running downhill and I would have to fetch it, one shoe on and one foot in a sock. (Talk about motion-out-of-control!) When my longest run reached

1.5 miles, I decided to make the switch to cheap Jack Purcell sneakers. The virginal New Balance trail-running shoes still remained in their box, untouched and unsullied. Plus, I wasn't doing any trail running. And so it went with my incremental progress as a jogger. Within two months, I was running three miles. It was time to head for the trails on nearby Mt. Tam.

During this period, I was also working on my own memoir *Return to Fitness,* reading articles about running, and talking with multisport coaches and health experts. One was my longtime friend, Dr. Phil Maffetone, who had coached several world-class endurance athletes, including six-time Hawaii Ironman triathlon champion Mark Allen. Maffetone also helped me regain my overall health by recommending a better diet. (And I stopped taking Advil.) He recommended that I run in flat-soled shoes, since he was convinced after treating patients and athletes for thirty years that the modern running shoe was the leading cause of most foot, calf, knee, and even hip injuries. "Buy your running shoes at Walmart, the cheapest and flattest you can find, " he told me. "It's where I buy my shoes."

I listened carefully to Phil's advice on footwear, but I felt as if I were sitting in on a talk given by a member of the Flat Earth Society. Why then did most running shoes have thickly cushioned footbeds, beefy soles, and monster heels? I thought back to the pair of Mizunos that successfully took me through the second Ironman. I had been averaging between fifteen and twenty-five miles a week of running. They definitely satisfied the criteria as built-up, over-supportive running shoes. Yet I never seemed to get injured; or maybe that had something to do with the cross-training rewards I accrued from biking and swimming.

Nor did I pay a moment's notice to running form. I just ran. I didn't care where or how my feet hit the ground. But during my fitness return, I happened to come across an article that referenced a widely publicized 1999 study by Dr. Steven Robbins, a biomechanics expert then at the McGill University Centre for Studies in Aging in Montreal, who suggested that expensive running shoes weren't worth the money and may even increase your risk of injury. Robbins also made the rather provocative claim that athletic shoes should be classified as "safety hazards" rather than "protective devices."

I gradually began to rethink my position on running shoes. On the big day I finally decided to go trail running, I found the New Balance shoebox, removed the shoes, laced them up, walked a few steps, then stopped. Something just didn't feel right. Or more precisely, my feet couldn't feel the floor because the shoes had too much padding and trread. If these shoes deprived my feet of any real kinesthetic awareness of the wooden floor, then I wouldn't be able to sense any of the roots, ruts, and rocks along the trail. Was this cushy desensitization going to ultimately help or hurt my running? So I did something radical. I slipped off the shoes, put them back in the box, and hoped that LL Bean would issue a refund. (They later did.) I ran instead in the Purcells, knowing that a flat, unsupported shoe would at least keep me out of trouble on the trails, because that had always been my foremost worry about getting back in shape after a decade of zero running—the fear of an injury, which would lead to permanently falling off the fitness wagon.

The five-mile trail run went fine. Afterwards, I phoned a friend in Colorado who is a hard-core mountain runner and world-champion pack-burro racer (the sport is so small that there are less than 200 racers) and asked for his opinion on the best trail-running shoes. "Go with the Nike Frees he told me. Best Nike shoe since the Pegasus"—which, as I mentioned earlier, was my first real running shoe. This conversation occurred in the spring of 2009. I had yet to read *Born to Run*, nor did I even know that such a book existed. After hunting around for an hour on the web, I found a pair of Nike Free 5.0s in my size on Zappos.com. I bought two pairs, as they were now discontinued. Several of the reviewer comments mentioned that they tended to fit a bit snug, so I went up a half-size. When the shoes arrived at my home, I removed both of the inner-sole liners. That was something Maffetone told me to do. "The less there is between your foot and the ground, the better off you are."

I immediately fell in love with the Frees. Their super-flexible, deep-channeled, sturdy foamlike tread encouraged my wide foot to land on its mid-section rather than heel. I felt lighter on my feet, as if I was leaning forward, with a bit more spring in the stride, encouraging my body to keep moving forward. Since I ran tortoise-slow—days of running sub-eight-minute miles were long gone—I cherished and appreciated what my body was allowing me to accomplish in a relaxed, aerobic state. I considered my running to be more like loping, an homage to Paleo man. Loping seemed like an agreeable compromise between jogging and running. I told friends, "Slow is the new fast."

The Nike Frees were the only running shoes I used for over a year and 750 miles. I wore them for my solo half-marathon run to the top of 2,500-foot Mount Tam that capped my triumphant return to fitness.

I ran another 500 miles in the Frees before I began to experiment with other types of "minimalist" footwear. By then, I had launched a running blog called *Zero Drop* and started to receive new minimalist running shoes from footwear companies.

Unlike Pete, I don't have a shoe addiction. My current footwear rotation is limited to only several brands. But I no longer run in the Frees. Why? As I progressed to a more natural running style, I no longer felt that I needed their extra cushiony support. I was learning to use my own lower legs as built-in shock absorbers. Maybe one day, I will go all the way to barefoot running. But I'm not there yet, and I see little reason to rush things. Running has become so damn enjoyable.

It's also easy to understand why converts to minimalist and barefoot-style running shoes have become passionate about less-is-more footwear. If *Born to Run* helped to initiate many of the changes we are currently seeing in the running world, we still have a very long way to go before a uniform consensus indeed emerges. Maybe it never will, because the various running and footwear camps seem as polarized and contentious as political factions. But there's one undeniable fact: Runners everywhere feel reborn. They have become interested in what happens when they run. It's no longer a matter of simply putting in the miles. It's now a question of footwear and form.

So let's begin our journey together . . . how our species first evolved as runners.

CHAPTER 1

⸎

The Evolution of Running in Humans

It has been said that the love of the chase is an inherent delight
in man—a relic of an instinctive passion.

—Charles Darwin

"You're going to ruin your knees!" How often do runners hear that gibe made by non-runners who feel compelled to criticize their exercise habit? Probably too numerous to even count. Unfortunately, the "ruined knee" comment is usually made by those who fail to consider the many positive health benefits of regular exercise, not to mention the fact that the weak muscles, fragile bones, and excess body fat that are associated with a sedentary lifestyle are likely to be far more damaging to one's joints than logging a few miles out on the road. And if you've managed to injure yourself while running, you'll often hear these same annoying busybodies make the specious claim that "humans just aren't built to run long distances!"

These naysayers live in the dark. Humans are spectacular long-distance runners, despite the toll that inactivity and poor nutrition have taken on a large swath of modern, developed society. We are a species that evolved to be physically active, and one that evolved to travel long distances on foot by walking, and yes, by running. So how did we develop this running prowess, and why is being inactive really the most unnatural thing a person can do?

The Origin of *Homo sapiens*

The human body evolved under a very different set of conditions than it is exposed to today. Our ancestral line split from that leading to the chimpanzee about 5 to 8 million years ago, when ape-like creatures climbed down from the trees of the African forests and began to spend more time on the ground. Initially, their diet was probably not dissimilar to that of modern tree-dwelling primates like the chimpanzee (with which we share about 98 percent genetic similarity). Chimps feed primarily on ripe fruits and other vegetable matter, using the energy provided from their high quality, carbohydrate rich food sources to fuel their gregarious and sociable behavior. However, in addition to their heavy intake of plant matter, chimps are also known to incorporate insects into their diet as an additional source of protein—you've probably seen the nature documentaries showing chimpanzees "fishing" for underground termites with a long stick. Furthermore, chimps on occasion are known to conduct communal hunts, typically targeting small mammals like colobus monkeys in the forest canopy. Chimps are therefore technically omnivores, just as most humans are today.

If the chimpanzee diet was potentially representative of our first ground-dwelling ancestors' diet, one can then hypothesize that some amount of meat was already part of the gustatory picture. However, life on the ground was very different from that in the trees, and as climate change converted this ancestral environment from tropical forests to savannah woodlands, adaptation was necessary for survival. Over time, and with the help of natural selection, our distant ancestors became more effective at bipedal locomotion. Indeed, fossilized footprints from 3.6 million years ago at Laetoli, Tanzania, indicate that *Australopithecus afarensis*, the species of which the famous "Lucy" skeleton belongs, was capable of bipedal walking. But mode of locomotion wasn't the only thing that began to change. Their digestive tract, jaws, and teeth became smaller as they developed the ability to process and cook food—soft, cooked food requires far less time spent chewing, and is much easier to digest than tough plant matter or raw meat. In fact, the relatively greater effort required to process, chew, and digest raw muscle explains in part why many carnivores will target fatty, soft organs like the intestines and brains of their prey before going after muscle. In addition to a more streamlined digestive system, our ancestors' brains began to enlarge—a higher quality, more easily digestible diet allowed for energy that previously would have been directed to gut development and digestion to be directed toward the development of a larger brain. A bigger brain would in turn have been advantageous for more effective tracking and hunting. They also began to use crude stone tools, and there's clear evidence that *Homo habilis* from roughly 2.5 million years ago was butchering flesh from animal bones.

That's not to say that our ancestors were pure carnivores—foraging, gathering, scavenging, and hunting for a variety of food types was likely the norm, as it is today with some modern hunter-gatherer tribes. Given the obvious importance of food to survival, physical traits that enhanced the ability of our ancestors to succeed at any type of food-acquiring behavior in this new environment were critical and would have been heavily favored by natural selection. Under evolutionary theory, it follows that these traits would have been more likely to have been passed on to subsequent generations, and as our bodies changed over time, our ability to acquire food in this new habitat improved.

By about 1.9 million years ago *Homo erectus* arrived on the scene, and based on fossil remains it appears to have been characterized by many of the anatomical traits that make modern humans both excellent walkers and runners. In an interview with *All Things Considered* host Jacki Lyden on National Public Radio, Harvard University primatologist Richard Wrangham described *Homo erectus* as "a species about our size . . . and the first one, one might say, that could walk down a street in a modern city and go into a store and get some clothes off the peg." In other words, they looked a lot like us. The combination of a developed brain and endurance on foot presumably allowed *Homo erectus* to effectively hunt prey in order to obtain the high-quality nutrients in animal meat. Fossil evidence clearly indicates that *Homo erectus* was a skilled enough hunter to have killed and eaten large, adult mammals that shared its habitat.

Evolutionary anthropologist Dr. Daniel Lieberman is professor and chairman of the Human Evolutionary Biology Department at Harvard University, and a curator at the Peabody Museum of Archaeology and Ethnology in Cambridge, Massachusetts. He's spent much of his career studying skeletal remains of ancestral humans, with a particular interest in the evolution of the human head, as well as the evolutionary origins of human distance running capabilities (he also happens to be a marathon runner himself). Given his in-depth knowledge of ancestral human behavior, we asked Lieberman to reconstruct a day in the life of *Homo erectus* and to comment in particular on the importance of meat in their diet:

> *We know that they were hunter-gatherers. Every day they would have had to go out hunting and foraging. Women probably gathered mostly. Men probably did a combination of foraging and hunting, and that meant that they probably walked long distances every day and occasionally ran. They probably climbed trees and dug holes for tubers—it's actually fairly hard work.*
>
> *Adult* Homo erectus *females were probably the most energetically constrained. The typical female* Homo erectus *would likely have been either pregnant or lactating most of the time, and she'd also probably have infants in tow. It's hard to establish how dependent they might have been, but they probably matured more rapidly than human infants. Given this, a typical* Homo erectus *female would need to take in at least 2000–4000 calories per day, with the higher end of that scale more likely for a pregnant or lactating female. It's a huge challenge for a hunter-gatherer to take in 4000 calories in a day—we think of it as trivial in our modern world of domesticated foods, but none of that existed back then. There had to be food sharing and some kind of food processing—bashing things up with rocks and the like. Meat would have been a very important part of the diet because you couldn't get that kind of energy effectively or efficiently without some reliance on meat—we know that from the archaeological record. So they probably were hunter-gatherers, maybe not exactly like today's hunter-gatherers, but the essence of hunter-gatherer way of life must have existed back then.*

Meat was clearly a high value resource for *Homo erectus* as its caloric density contributed not only to the survival of healthy adults but also helped to nourish the developing offspring and those who cared for them. As a result, it's not surprising that *Homo erectus* is generally considered to be the first truly efficient hominid hunter.

Modern man, *Homo sapiens*, first appears in the fossil record about 200,000 years ago and provided us with the body that we have today— a tall, big-brained, omnivorous, bipedal, long-legged mammal that can

THE EVOLUTION OF RUNNING IN HUMANS • 5

outrun just about any other animal on the planet over a long distance. We are a product of our ancestry, and looking back in time in a bit more detail can provide clues about how our earliest relatives obtained the meat that was so important to their survival.

Enter the Running Man

So how did they do it? How were early humans like *Homo erectus* able to kill animals that in many cases were larger, stronger, and faster than them? Despite archaeological evidence confirming that meat was part of our ancestral diet extending back at least 2.5 million years, other discoveries indicate that stone-tipped spears did not appear until around 300,000 years ago. More advanced projectile weaponry like bows and arrows have only been around for some 50,000 years. Determining how our ancestors obtained their meat can read like a detective story, with partial clues pointing to likely scenarios. Unlike lions and other top-of-the-food chain predators on the African savannah that can take down prey with their short-burst speed, brute strength, and vicious claws and teeth, humans are slow and wimpy and would have little hope of taking down a large antelope via ambush with their bare hands.

One solution to hunting without on-board armaments like razor-sharp claws or piercing teeth is to build weaponry from resources found in the environment. However, long before early man could take advantage of projectile attacks using weapons like spear throwers, bows and arrows, or hunting rifles, he had to hunt with far more rudimentary and less effective weapons. According to Lieberman, "the most lethal weapon available to a *Homo erectus* hunter would have been a sharpened wooden stick or a club." Of course, the use of such simple weaponry would have required fairly close proximity to the prey in order to make a kill. "I wouldn't want to see anybody try to go up to an animal and shove a sharpened stick into it from close quarters," Lieberman continues. "You'd be much better off being a vegetarian! One kick, one graze from its horns and your evolutionary fitness has gone down considerably. We know from the ethnographic record that modern hunter-gatherers are very loathe to get close to big animals. It's dangerous! So they use projectiles, but projectiles weren't invented until recently." Therein lies the mystery—for some 1.5 to 1.6 million years from the appearance of *Homo erectus* to the appearance of the stone-tipped spear, our ancestors hunted and killed animals with nothing more than simple wooden weapons. How the heck did they do it?

The answer, some scientists and anthropologists think, is by running. Not fast, mind you. Olympic sprinters would have trouble chasing down even the slowest of prey on the savannah at an all-out pace. When Usain Bolt set the world-record in the 100 meters, it was calculated that his average speed was 23 miles per hour, which is slightly less than half the top land-speed of a lion or gazelle. Rather, according to hypotheses put forth by Harvard's Lieberman and evolutionary biologists David Carrier and Dennis Bramble of the University of Utah, our ancestors evolved traits that allowed them to excel at slow-paced endurance running rather than high-speed sprinting.

The endurance hunting or "Running Man" hypothesis put forth by these three researchers emphasized that our ancestors excelled at a food acquisition method known as persistence hunting. This involves capturing prey by running them to exhaustion, at which point the spent animal can be approached and killed with ease and little danger to the hunter. The idea that a human could run down an antelope that is many times larger and many times faster may seem far-fetched, but the reality is that the practice is still employed by isolated modern tribes such as the Kalahari Bushmen in Africa. In fact, a modern-day persistence hunt was featured in a nature documentary released in 2003 by the BBC.

In an episode of the BBC video series *The Life of Mammals*, Sir David Attenborough narrates as a group of Kalahari Bushmen carry out a persistence hunt of a full-grown kudu in the mid-day sun. Seen on the video are three hunters who specifically target an enormous adult male kudu. They believe that its large size and heavy horns will make it tire more quickly than smaller kudus. The hunters alternate periods of walking and running as they track and chase, carefully attempting to separate the bull from its pack and keep it moving, never allowing it to rest and cool down. As they sense the Kudu beginning to overheat under the unforgiving sun of the open savannah, the "runner" (who we feel obliged to point out was wearing cheap sneakers) takes over, leaving his fellow hunters behind as he takes on the burden of the final chase. After hours of relentless pursuit, the weary kudu seems to be running out of gas, its legs unsteady, and its breathing shallow and fast. As the "runner" moves within striking distance, the kudu makes a feeble attempt to flee, but instead its legs buckle and it crumples helplessly to the sun-baked, dusty earth. It has no hope of escape, nor any energy to put up a fight—its threatening horns are no longer a risk to the still-nimble hunter. The "runner" approaches, and with a quick throw of his spear dispatches his prey.

If these modern hunters provide a reasonable representation of how our ancestors carried out a persistence hunt, then it shows very clearly what ancestral endurance running might have looked like. The hunters used more of a walk-run approach to the hunt, and even when running, it was by no means similar to the all-out pace for 26.2 miles that many modern runners view as the pinnacle of running performance. In many ways, the style exhibited by the Bushmen has a lot more in common with the run-walk method advocated by well-known marathon coach Jeff Galloway, or the style employed by modern ultramarathoners, who will typically walk up steep hills, blaze down declines, and employ a moderate pace on the flats. (Even kids don't tend to run long distances at fast, or even moderate, pace. They intersperse jogging, sprinting, and walking almost continuously when playing outdoors, and they rarely stop moving. This gets to the notion that juveniles of any animal tend to play with behaviors that are critical to their ultimate lifestyle. For example, watch puppies wrestling or kittens play-hunting. A kid runs more like a persistence hunter than a marathoner intent on setting a PR.)

Ultimately, the slow and steady approach brought the hunter to his quarry, and brought meat back to his kin. When Lieberman was asked how frequent persistence hunting might have occurred among early humans, he candidly responded, "Nobody really has the foggiest idea. But we have to come up with an explanation for how and why humans started endurance running. I have a hard time imagining that it wasn't an important way of bringing home the bacon a few million years ago. I've been racking my brain for twenty years, literally, and I still can't come up with another explanation."

Lieberman, however, offers an interesting viewpoint explaining the differences between the style of endurance running critical to the survival success of the ancestral persistence hunter and that of the modern marathon runner. For many modern runners, completion of a marathon is a defining moment and a source of immense personal pride; running a marathon quickly enough to meet the bar for qualification into a hal-lowed race like the Boston Marathon is a badge of running success nearly without equal. However, running 26.2 miles as fast as possible was cer-tainly not likely a regular occurrence for the persistence hunter. "If you actually look at the data, they're (persistence hunters) not running the entire time," says Lieberman. "They're running part of the time and walk-ing part of the time. It's a combination of chasing and tracking. The idea that you should run and not stop—it's kind of nuts! I don't think any persistence hunter probably ever did that, or at least not very often. They probably could do it, but they didn't, at least not from the data I've seen. So yes, the idea that you can put on a pair of shoes and run 26.2 miles as fast as you can without stopping is really kind of a bizarre thing. We've kind of turned a human capability into something different, which is a classic human thing to do."

In other words, most modern runners share little in common with the ancestral hunter on the African savannah. Modern runners log work-outs, track splits, blare fast-paced music through earbuds, and wear GPS watches that spit out pace and heart rate in order to monitor speed and exertion, all in an effort to maybe go a few seconds or minutes faster at the next race. Training gadgets are fun for sure, but one can't help but wonder if all of this focus on speed really distracts from what humans are really good at, which is running slow and long. It also might be a big reason why runners often get hurt—running with a single-minded focus on setting a PR can cause them to push their limits against their better judgment and prevent them from heeding warning signs when they appear. It can be a worthwhile experiment to ditch the distractions at least once in awhile and simply run easy and for fun—no watch, no music, no heart rate monitor. Just you, your surroundings, and the road or trail down below.

Despite the appeal of the persistence-hunting hypothesis, particu-larly among distance runners who look at it as evolutionary validation for what many non-runners view as a strange and self-destructive sport, there are some who dispute the idea that persistence hunting was a regu-larly employed behavior among early humans. Some suggest that perhaps early man ambushed prey by throwing wooden spears down from trees at animals that passed underneath. Lieberman responds, "Ambush hunting could have occurred, in fact I'm sure it probably occurred occasionally for small animals. But for big animals? You'd have to be nuts! Furthermore, if you try to throw a sharpened wooden stick at a big animal like a kudu, it just bounces off the hide. What kills an animal is not the hole, it's the lacerations caused by the point inside the animal. So until those stone tools were invented, we didn't have the kinds of modern methods that some are thinking about to hunt and effectively kill animals." Furthermore, even if an early human hunter managed to stab and wound an antelope with a wooden spear, running might still have been required if the wounded animal took off and the hunter wanted to track it and either finish it off or retrieve the carcass before it was taken by competing predators in the vicinity. That's not to say that this didn't happen or that ambush wasn't a part of our ancestral hunting strategy, just that alternative methods could have also been used that exploited the hunter's physiological strengths, one of which was his ability to run long in the heat of day.

Another recent argument that has been made against the persistence-hunting hypothesis was that if early humans hunted prey by running them down, fossils of animals killed and eaten by these individuals should be similar to those targeted by modern running animals—namely, the young, the sick, and the old. However, fossil data suggest that *Homo erectus* selectively targeted prime adults, which anthropologists Henry Bunn of the University of Wisconsin-Madison and Travis Pickering of the University of the Witwatersrand in South Africa put forth as evidence refuting the endurance running hypothesis in a 2010 paper in the journal *Quaternary Research*. When asked about this, Lieberman responded, "Modern hunter-gatherers state very bluntly that they pick the biggest animals to hunt because they know that they overheat the fastest. So the fact that they found prime aged adults is actually confirmatory evidence for our theory." In other words, large animals have more muscle, which generates more heat, and less body surface relative to their size across which to dissipate that heat. The upshot: if you're going to run down and kill an animal by causing it to overheat, pick the biggest, heaviest one you can find.

Although the continuing existence of persistence hunting in modern tribes such as the Kalahari Bushmen suggests that it has a long history and has been retained because it is an effective hunting technique, it may not be the only way ancestral humans utilized their endurance to fill their bellies. An alternative strategy for which endurance running may have been equally important is scavenging. "If you ever go to Africa you'll notice that carcasses are not just hanging out on the savannah. They get eaten almost instantly," says Lieberman. "They're such high-value resources. Hyenas get there, jackals get there, vultures. There's a reason why carnivores run—they run to hunt, but they also have to run to compete. So running might have also been very important for scavenging as well."

Early human scavenging likely involved running to feast on fresh carcasses before they were eaten by the other garbage-collecting animals. Thus, scavenging was another situation in which running would have been important. Our ancestors could have used signs like circling vultures on the horizon as a homing beacon to find fresh kills, which would surely have called in competing scavengers that needed to be beaten to the prize. Quick arrival at the carcass might have yielded a healthy portion of meat, or at least some bones that could be cracked open to access the fatty marrow located inside.

Both Bramble and Lieberman suggest that endurance scavenging may even have been a first step in the evolution of the running man. According to Lieberman, in evolution "things generally don't just happen instantaneously; there's typically a transition, and I can well imagine that running might have initially been favored by natural selection for animals that could scavenge a little bit better, and then those animals had some ability to hunt a little bit better. These things are never simple stories."

Regardless of whether early man's primary strategy for obtaining meat was persistence hunting, endurance scavenging, or whether he used some combination of these along with other methods like ambush hunting, it is quite plausible that being able to run long was of potentially significant benefit to our ancestors, and bringing home a bounty of meat would be a huge benefit to both hunter and tribe. Individuals who could hunt well without dying in the process were better at passing along their genes and ensuring the survival of their kin, and over hundreds of thousands of years natural selection produced a body that was capable of carrying out an endurance hunt quite effectively. This is, in most respects, a body that is identical in its fundamental anatomy and physiology to the one you possess as you read this, and it is a body that instills in you a great deal of potential: with a bit of endurance training, you can outrun the vast majority of other species on this planet over a long distance.

How Do Humans Stack Up as Runners?

There is little argument that humans as a species are amazingly good endurance runners. This trait suggests that running ability must have been favored by natural selection at some point in our evolutionary history. In fact, we may just be among the best of all animals when it comes to endurance running. This realization is not new—legendary ultrarunner Arthur Newton emphasized human distance running prowess in his 1935 book *Running*:

Just compare the size and development of a man's legs (as against his physique) with any of the fastest running animals. The greyhound type of dog may be more advanced, but the horse and ordinary dog are almost certainly less so. This means that for goodness only knows how many thousands of years men must have been more competent distance runners than the majority of animals. Since the size and development remain, it is just as certain that the ability is not entirely lost, but is only latent and can be more or less worked up at any time.

As Newton recognized decades ago, what humans lack in pure speed, they more than make up for in their ability to run long distances at a slow, sustained pace. For this reason, we are one of a select few species that can actually run a 26.2-mile footrace without stopping. However, depending on temperature and conditions, we would have competition for the top spot in an inter-species endurance running competition. For example, Alaskan sled-racing dogs are specifically bred to run one hundred or more miles per day, day in and day out, never seeming to tire of the exertion. In fact, during the annual Iditarod race in Alaska, teams of twelve to sixteen dogs pull sled and musher over 1100 miles from Anchorage to Nome in as few as eight or nine days. Sled dogs are true physiological marvels with a huge aerobic capacity, an ability to rapidly adapt to exercise related stresses, and a remarkable ability to burn fat and spare glycogen in a way that champion human marathoners could only dream of. However, despite the many unique aspects of their physiology, they require cold temperatures to perform their incredible feats of endurance. In fact, sled dogs often spend much of the summer resting for this very reason—kind of like a canine off-season. Just like with your pet pooch, sled dogs don't tolerate heat well, and running them hard on a hot day is downright dangerous. Match a sled dog up against a well-conditioned human at the starting line of a marathon on a hot day, and you'd be wise to place your bets on the human to be the first, and perhaps only, racer to reach the finish line.

In a 2007 paper in the journal *Sports Medicine* titled "*The Evolution of Marathon Running Capabilities in Humans*," authors Daniel Lieberman and Dennis Bramble stated that "for marathon-length distances, humans can outrun almost all other mammals and can sometimes outrun even horses, especially when it is hot." Yet, if you asked the average person if they thought a human could outrun a horse in a long distance race, the answer would most likely be a resounding "no." In fact, they'd probably consider the idea of a human being able to outrun a horse at any distance to be preposterous, even if the horse was carrying a rider. However, if you happen to be an elite marathoner and the race covers 22 rugged miles in the Welsh town of Llanwrtyd Wells, there's a decent chance that you could emerge victorious. In fact, this exact result has happened twice recently at the annual Man versus Horse Marathon.

Started in 1980, the Man versus Horse Marathon was initiated as a result of a challenge proposed in a pub (seemingly the location where all matches of this kind begin). Over the past 30 years, the race has grown to include over 600 runners and 40 horses. Perhaps the most impressive thing about this particular race is that in 2004, after almost 25 years of equine domination, the race was won by a human. Not only did Huw Lobb win the race in 2:05:19, he defeated the runner-up, a horse named Kay Bee Jay, by over two full minutes. When asked by the BBC News what he would do with the £25,000 in prize money he earned, Lobb responded "the first thing that I will do with the money is buy myself some decent training shoes." It would be interesting to know what kind of training shoes are favored by a man who can outrun a horse . . .

Lobb's victory for the human side was repeated in 2007, when Florian Holzinger won the race with a time of 2:20:30, eleven minutes ahead of the nearest horse. In 2008 and 2009, a horse named Dukes Touch of Fun reclaimed the title for the equine side, and in 2010 Sly Dai made it a three-peat for the horses. In response to Dukes Touch of Fun's 2008 victory, her owner, John McFarlane, told the *Telegraph* that "we cut it a bit fine but we have proved that horse is superior to human . . . she deserves a good rest and some extra carrots now." Although a human has only won twice, Huw Lobb's victorious time from 2004 has not been bested since by either species.

Though the Man vs. Horse Marathon might be little more than a curiosity among long-distance races, one of the biggest and most competitive events in the modern ultramarathon circuit has its roots in horse racing. The Western States Endurance Run, a 100-mile race across the Sierra Nevada mountains of Northern California, is one of the oldest and most prestigious ultra trail events. However, it was originally an equestrian event called the Western States Trail Ride, not a race among fleet-footed humans possessing seemingly superhuman endurance. In 1974, Gordon Ainsleigh, a big, bearded hulk of a man, faced a predicament—his horse had come up lame during the race the previous year. Rather than risk a repeat occurrence with his unreliable horse, Ainsleigh started training with the intent to tackle the race on foot. Ainsleigh made good on his plan, entered the race without his horse, and he wound up beating the 24-hour time limit set for the riders. In doing so, he earned a coveted silver buckle and became the first human to complete this storied race on foot. Ainsleigh's successful completion of what had historically been a competition among horses shows once again that humans really are excellent distance runners even when compared to one of the best endurance running animals on the planet. Even more remarkable is the speed of today's elite ultrarunners. The men's record at the Western States 100 is 15 hours and 7 minutes, set by Geoff Roes in 2010; Ann Trason, who won the event a mind-boggling fourteen times, established the women's record of 17 minutes and 34 minutes in 1994.

The Anatomy of an Endurance Running Specialist

What is it about the human body makes it ideally suited to run for long distances? The short answer is that humans possess a number of anatomical and physiological traits not present in their nearest living primate relatives (chimpanzees). Unlike humans, chimpanzees are primarily arboreal creatures who spend much of their time in trees. Just as humans are not particularly good at swinging around in the forest canopy, chimps don't move very well when they do come down to the ground. In fact, researchers have trained chimps to walk on a treadmill while measuring their oxygen consumption (a proxy for energy expenditure) with a face mask, and have shown that walking is as much as 75 percent more metabolically costly when compared to humans. In other words, humans are far more efficient than chimps when it comes to over-ground walking. What's more, though a chimp on the ground can run fast for short distances, endurance running in chimpanzees is unheard of (though the mental image is kind of amusing).

What are the specific traits that separate man from chimp that facilitate movement over long distances on the ground? In a 2004 paper published in the journal *Nature*, Dennis Bramble and Daniel Lieberman identified human traits in four basic areas that seem to have evolved due to their benefit for running. They grouped these traits into four categories:

1. Energetics. The human running gait differs from walking in a number of ways. One critical difference is that running involves a much greater degree of compliance of the limbs—in other words, whereas walking involves a relatively straight leg with less flex at the knee, the leg during running essentially acts like a spring. It compresses when it hits the ground, and extends as it pushes off—this is accomplished by a much greater degree of flexion and extension at each joint. A benefit of running is that as muscles and tendons are stretched, they store elastic energy like a rubber band, and that energy is then returned when these tissues shorten, contributing to propulsion as the leg straightens back out.

Compared to chimpanzees, humans are endowed with a specialized set of springy tendons and ligaments in the legs and feet, prime examples of which are the Achilles tendon attaching the calf muscles to the heel, and the connective tissues that help to support the longitudinal arch of the foot. In chimpanzees the Achilles tendon is poorly developed, and the foot lacks a longitudinal arch—the feet and legs of chimpanzees are more suited to hanging from a tree branch than running on the ground. In a running human who lands on the forefoot, the Achilles tendon and attached calf musculature stretch as the heel comes down after initial ground contact is made in the area behind the base of the little toe. The calf muscles are actively contracting as they stretch during this process (this is known as an eccentric contraction), making the Achilles tendon more taut. The contracting calf muscles and taut Achilles pull upward on the calcaneus bone at the back of the heel, preventing the heel from coming down too fast and colliding hard with the ground. This process stores up energy in these tissues, and, incidentally, is likely the reason why runners who start running barefoot or in minimal shoes often find that their calves get very sore during the transition period—eccentric muscle contractions are more likely to cause delayed onset muscle soreness. As the heel lifts off the ground during push-off, the calf and Achilles shorten, and the previously stored energy is released—kind of like stretching a bungee cord and then letting one end go. In a study published in the journal *Nature* in 1987, Robert Ker of the University of Leeds and colleagues estimated that as much as 35 percent of the energy lost and regained during each running step is stored in the Achilles tendon and returned to the runner via elastic recoil.

A similar process occurs with the medial longitudinal arch of the foot. If you were to look at the skeletal foot of a chimpanzee, you would notice that it has no arch. Most humans, on the other hand, have a very distinct arch on the inner side of the foot—this is known as the medial longitudinal arch (there are several other arches, but we'll focus on this one for now). When the foot hits the ground, the arch compresses and flattens to some degree, and like the Achilles tendon, connective tissues and plantar muscles attached to the bony arch store elastic energy which is then returned during push-off. Estimates by Ker and colleagues, who obtained their data somewhat gruesomely by using machines to compress the arches of amputated human feet, suggest that the arch stores and returns as much as 17 percent of the energy required during a running step. Taken together, Bramble and Lieberman indicate that the "springs" in human legs and feet save one as much as 50 percent of the metabolic cost of running, and are one of the reasons why a chimp stands little chance of beating human in a long-distance footrace.

Another factor relating to human lower limb anatomy that has relevance to the endurance running hypothesis is that humans have longer legs than chimps, allowing for a longer stride length (though it should be noted that among humans, leg length is not a great predictor of stride length). Furthermore, the mass of the human lower leg and foot are relatively reduced. The human foot, according to Bramble and Lieberman, represents only 9 percent of total leg mass, whereas it contributes 14 percent of the leg mass in a chimp. Granted, long, skinny legs could also provide an advantage during walking, but the significance of a reduction of weight at the end of the leg is well known to any runner who has grown accustomed to running in ultra-light racing flats. Put on a pair of heavy training shoes and it feels like you are running with bricks on your feet! The more weight you put at the end of the leg, the more energy it will take to swing that leg while running. It's for the very same reason that it's easier to swing a golf club than it is to swing a sledge hammer. It's also the reason why nearly all of the animals that one thinks of as being good runners—dogs, horses, antelope, cheetahs—have long, skinny legs. Some of these animals have gone so far as to reduce the foot to a hoof—they essentially run on the tips of their toes. We're not advocating that anyone go out and try to run like a pirouetting ballerina, but it's interesting to consider that our toes are also considerably shorter than those of our modern primate cousins.

2. Stabilization. Human walking and running gaits differ in a number of ways. Aside from the obvious increase in speed and greater bending of the lower limb joints that characterize running, the running gait is also distinguished by the incorporation of a distinct "flight" or "aerial" phase. In walking, one foot always contacts the ground. In contrast, running can be modeled as a series of jumps from one foot to the other, with the flight phase being the time when the body is fully airborne between landings (incidentally, continuous contact of at least one foot with the ground is required of race-walking competitors—"loss of contact" is considered a violation because it indicates that the competitor is running rather than walking). Because of the more rapid and dynamic nature of the motions involved, as well as the fact running involves repeatedly leaping through the air and balancing on one foot during stance phase, it is harder to stabilize the body while running than it is to do so while walking, especially in bipeds. When your foot hits the ground during running, a braking effect occurs and without internal stabilization your body would tend to pitch forward and plunge face-first into the ground. This generally doesn't happen, mainly because humans have anatomical characteristics that confer a great deal of stability while running.

Among the traits that contribute to stabilization of the human body is the presence of a well-developed gluteus maximus that is mostly active while running (the gluteus maximus is the large muscle that makes up much of the mass of your butt). Chimps have a comparatively scrawny bum, and studies have shown that the gluteus maximus fires heavily during human running, but remains quiet during level walking. The big butt muscle helps to stabilize the trunk and maintain upright posture while running, but that's not all that this muscle does. It also slows the swing leg as it prepares for landing, helping to prevent overextension of the thigh. Even more importantly for a runner, the gluteus maximus functions to pull the thigh backward to provide forward propulsion as we run. Ever wonder why sprinters tend to have big muscular butts? That's because strong glutes are critical to being able to propel these runners forward as rapidly as possible when they run all-out. But, the gluteus maximus is important in assisting forward drive in slower-paced distance running as well—though an Olympic marathoner isn't likely to have a butt as big as an Olympic 100-meter sprinter, one can safely assume that it's quite a bit larger than the glutes of a chimp. Thus, given these critical functions, along with their lack of activity in walking, a plausible case can be made that the human's enlarged glutes seem to be an adaptation for running.

Further contributing to stabilization, humans also have a band of connective tissue called the nuchal ligament that attaches the upper vertebrae to the back of the skull—if you place your own fingers at the base of the bony bump on the back of your head and tilt your chin down to your chest, you will feel this ligament pop out. When you are running, this ligament helps to prevent your big brainy head from lolling about. The nuchal ligament is found in a number of other running animals such as dogs and horses, but is notably absent in chimps. Fossil evidence also suggests that it is missing in some of our early hominid ancestors (e.g., *Australopithecus*), and its presence in *Homo* may represent yet another adaptation in support of our more advanced bipedal capabilities.

If you think about the movement of your body as you run, you probably tend to focus on what your legs are doing. However, the motions of your torso and arms are also important to the biomechanics of running. As one leg extends forward, it causes rotation of the lower body that would tend, in turn, to twist the upper body in the same direction if it were not counteracted in some way—this is where arm swing comes into play. The arm on the opposite side of the body extends forward at the same time as the leg, and the correlated rotation of the torso counteracts the rotation of the lower body. Think of it this way—as you run, your lower body is tending to rotate in one direction as each leg moves forward. At the same time the upper body and arm rotate in the opposite direction. These opposite rotations cancel one another out and keep you moving forward in a straight line. But here's the key point: humans are much better able to do this than a chimpanzee, in part because they can rotate their torso largely independent of the pelvis and head. There are several reasons for this. First, when compared to chimps, the human waist is narrower and is characterized by greater separation between the pelvis and thorax. Second, human shoulders are relatively wider, which increases the counterbalancing effect of rotating the torso. And third, muscular connections between the human torso and head are dramatically reduced, allowing the head to gaze steadily forward as the torso and shoulders rotate back and forth underneath it. Taken together, all of these stabilizing adaptations allow humans to run forward steadily and upright in a more or less straight line, all the while retaining independent movement of the head so they scan the horizon or ground in front of them.

3. Skeletal Strength. Running is an inherently stressful activity for the human body. Every time you take a step while running, your foot collides with the ground with a force equivalent to approximately two to three times your body weight, which is roughly double the force applied during walking (scientists refer to these forces as ground reaction forces). Naturally, dealing with these collision forces requires mechanisms to help dissipate the force, otherwise the body would eventually begin to break down (as it does in runners who overtrain). The springy limbs discussed above are one critical way to reduce impact-related damage during running, but from a skeletal standpoint, humans also possess a number of adaptations for stress dissipation that appear to differentiate them from their more arboreal ancestors. One change that has occurred is the expansion of bony joint surfaces in places like the knee, hip and between the vertebrae in order to spread out the area over which force is applied during ground contact. The implications of how a broader joint surface can help with stress reduction can be understood by considering the difference between stepping on a pointy rock versus a flat stone. Force application by the pointy rock is tightly focused on one small area, which causes a great deal of focal pain, whereas force application is spread out when stepping on a flat stone, and thus it doesn't hurt at all. Better to have the joint surfaces behave more like flat stones than jagged rocks when they compress together during ground contact—the greater the size of the surface over which a given amount of force is applied, the less that is applied to any single location. Lieberman and Bramble point out that similar expansion of joint surfaces does not occur in the upper limbs of *Homo*, suggesting that the human's bipedal gait and the associated forces generated during contact of their feet with the ground may have created a situation in which broader joint surfaces in the lower body were favored by natural selection.

4. Thermoregulation. We now come to the final, and perhaps most important adaptation that allows humans to be exceptional endurance runners, and it has to do with their ability to effectively manage body temperature.

When an animal exercises, its contracting muscles generate heat. If heat accumulation continues unabated, core body temperature could rise to dangerous levels—a phenomenon known as hyperthermia. Risk of overheating during exercise, in turn, is heightened if the environmental temperature is high, as this creates unfavorable conditions for the offloading of heat to the outside environment. Hyperthermia can be life threatening, so effective cooling mechanisms are critical for an animal that is active during the heat of day.

Among quadrupedal (four-legged) mammals, panting is one of the most commonly employed mechanisms for dissipating excess heat—that's why a dog's tongue sticks way out when they run in warm weather. In panting, the moisture on the animal's tongue evaporates, thus helping to cool it down. However, an owner who takes his or her dog for a run on a hot summer day is placing the pet at great risk. The combination of external heat from the environment and internal heat generated by working muscles can combine to overwhelm its canine cooling mechanism and lead to rapid development of hyperthermia—the dog's tongue simply does not provide a large enough surface area for evaporative cooling, and most of its sweat glands are located around the pads of its feet. Dogs that are pushed too hard on a hot day often start frothing at the mouth, and can end up listless, or worse, dead. Unlike humans, dogs simply cannot handle running hard in the heat, and the same applies to most other quadrupeds as well.

From the perspective of a hunter, knowledge of the inferior cooling mechanisms employed by prey provides a distinct advantage—get a quadruped to run hard on a hot day and it will be forced into hyperthermia, thus making it an easy kill. A particularly effective way to initiate hyperthermia in a quadruped that cools by panting is by making it run at a gallop rather than a trot. Quadrupeds are efficient runners from a metabolic standpoint. In a now classic paper from a 1984 issue of the journal *Current Anthropology*, David Carrier wrote that "running humans expend about twice as much energy per unit mass as typical quadrupeds of the same size." Unlike bipedal humans (and ignoring sprinting), however, quadrupeds use multiple distinct gaits when they run, and these gaits pose certain constraints not experienced by running humans.

The quadruped endurance gait is known as a trot. A trot is when the animal runs via synchronized motion of opposite-side fore and hind limbs—the right forelimb moving forward and backward in synchrony with the left hind limb and so on. When an animal like a dog or antelope trots, it can breathe freely and can cool its body effectively via panting. In order to run faster, however, quadrupeds must transition to a gait known as a gallop (or a slower form of galloping known as a canter). A gallop is a much more dynamic gait in which the synchrony between opposite-side limbs as seen in a trot is lost. Galloping involves extension of the back as the hind limbs push off, which expands the torso and allows the animal to breathe in. As the animal impacts the ground on its forelimbs, the back arches and its guts push forward against its diaphragm and lungs, forcing it to exhale. Watch a dog playing fetch and you will typically see these two gaits demonstrated quite clearly—it will typically gallop rapidly when it chases a thrown ball, and it will trot back to its owner with the ball in its mouth. As a result of this pattern of movement, respiration in galloping animals is tightly tied to their movements—they inhale as they take off and the lungs expand, and exhale when the lungs compress when they land. As a result, they can take only one breath per take-off/landing cycle. This makes cooling via panting very inefficient in a galloping animal, and therefore quadrupeds cannot sustain a gallop for very long without overheating.

Given the above factors, if one wanted to drive a quadruped into hyperthermia, an effective mechanism would be to get it to gallop on a hot day. Humans have a secret weapon that allows them to do just this—the ability to sweat. Some other animals also use sweat as a cooling mechanism (for example, horses, camels, and kangaroos), but humans have an additional advantage—we are largely hairless (well, most of us). This makes evaporative heat loss via sweating much more effective. When you run, you sweat, often profusely. And when you sweat, you cool down due to evaporation of moisture from the skin surface. Combined with the fact that man's long springy legs and metabolic engine allowed him to sustain endurance running speeds that exceed the trot-gallop transition for many quadrupeds, the ability to more effectively dissipate heat made early man a deadly hunter on the African savannah. Says Daniel Lieberman, "The whole point of a persistence hunt is to make the animal gallop. Natural selection didn't care if you ran 5-minute miles or 10-minute miles, all it cared about was getting that animal to gallop for more than ten to fifteen minutes at a time." In other words, humans didn't need to run fast; they just needed to run fast enough. All the hunter needed to do was find a target, keep it moving at a gallop for as long as possible, and minimize the time it had to rest and cool itself—this is the essence of a persistence hunt. Do this for long enough, and the animal overheats, collapses to the ground, and is incapable of fending off a close range attack. In other words, the beast has become dinner.

⌀⊗⌀

Given the unique attributes of human anatomy, it's unfortunate that running as a survival mechanism is no longer necessary or required in most of the modern world. Persistence hunting, these days, means patiently (or rather impatiently) waiting in long checkout lines at the supermarket or fast-food drive-thru. Yet, for the millions who do run, from the recreational jogger to elite racer, there is something else going on that appears to negate the outcomes of natural selection—at least in terms of long-distance running. It presents a rather strange predicament or riddle—humans evolved to run, but they just can't seem to go for a long time or with any consistency without getting hurt. The running human has become the injured human, and the search for the reason is complex, vexing, and seemingly never-ending.

⌀⊗⌀

CHAPTER 2

❧

Running Injuries: Why They Happen

Train, don't strain.—Arthur Lydiard

Pain. Virtually every runner has experienced it at some point and in some form. You might be blazing down the road, or bounding down a rocky dirt trail, and something starts to feel off. It might be a dull ache on the side of your knee, a sharp pull at the back of your ankle, or a strange feeling of tension in the arch of your foot—somewhere in the lower half of your body something is unhappy. You try to ignore it, but with every step your anxiety grows along with the feeling that something is genuinely wrong. Your heart starts to pound a bit harder. The dull ache starts to slowly morph into a shooting pain. You don't know why the pain is there, but now there's no denying it. You fear that if you continue, you may do lasting damage—your worst fear is that the damage may be significant enough that it will relegate you to the couch. You tremble at the thought of not being able to run. So you stop, limp home, and start cursing your damaged body. You are officially injured, you don't know why, and you aren't sure what to do next.

If the human species has evolved to run, then why do runners so often get hurt? That's really the billion-dollar question that runners want answered. Plantar fasciitis, iliotibial band syndrome (ITBS), Achilles tendinopathy, stress fracture, patellofemoral pain syndrome—if you're a runner you've likely heard these names before, and some of them might bring back painful memories of times when you had been forced to sit on the sidelines. What's more, many of these conditions can be nagging and frustratingly difficult to overcome. You probably know a runner who has dealt with a case of plantar fasciitis that lingered for months with no let up. Perhaps that runner is you? The reality is that most of us know, and are quite possibly surrounded by, broken runners. They have all sustained injuries through years of running that have forced them to either contemplate or actually give up the sport they love so much. What can be done to help these runners? Are there strategies that runners can employ to reduce their chance of getting hurt? Should they just quit running altogether since the risk of injury is so high? Let's start our discussion of injury by addressing this last question—why should we run?

Why We Should Run

Imagine for a moment that you went to see your doctor for your annual physical examination. After a routine workup, your physician told you they could give you a prescription that, if followed, would confer all of the following benefits:

- Lower risk of early death
- Lower risk of coronary artery disease
- Lower risk of stroke
- Lower risk of high blood pressure
- Lower risk of adverse blood lipid profile
- Lower risk of type 2 diabetes
- Lower risk of metabolic syndrome
- Lower risk of colon cancer
- Lower risk of breast cancer
- Prevention of weight gain
- Weight loss, particularly when combined with reduced calorie intake
- Improved cardiorespiratory and muscular fitness
- Prevention of falls
- Reduced depression
- Better cognitive function (for older adults)

Would you accept this prescription? We're guessing that you would—who wouldn't? You ask the doctor how much the prescription costs—you suspect it's not going to be cheap. Surely any pharmaceutical company that was able to produce a pill conferring all of these benefits would have on its hands a money-maker of astronomical proportions! Your doctor's response: "It's free." Okay, that's a bit of a surprise, but what about side effects? "Maybe some muscle soreness, excessive sweating, and an increased risk of musculoskeletal injury," replies the doctor. "Oh, and it requires that you give up a bit of your free time." "What is this wonder drug," you ask? Your doctor's response is simple and consists of one word: "exercise." The miracle prescription is physical activity.

In 2008, the U.S. Department of Health and Human Services (HHS) published a report called *The 2008 Physical Activity Guidelines for Americans*. In the report, the HHS states that "only a few lifestyle choices have as large an effect on mortality as physical activity" and indicates that scientific research has shown strong evidence for an association between all of the health benefits listed above and regular physical activity. What's more, the cost in terms of time to reduce your overall risk of premature death via getting active is fairly minimal—90 minutes per week of moderate to vigorous physical activity is all it takes to see a reduction. It would be hard to argue that all of the above aren't a worthwhile tradeoff to the risk of suffering an injury while exercising—indeed, the HHS report states openly that "the benefits of physical activity . . . outweigh the risk of injury." What's amazing though is that the prescription of exercise, which has been proven effective at reducing our risk of succumbing to some of the biggest killers in modern society, is so often turned down. If it were a pill, it would be wildly successful, but because exercise requires us to get up and move—to use our legs, hearts, and lungs as nature intended—most Americans let the advice to get physically active enter one ear and slip right out the other. They make excuses—exercise hurts, it takes too much time—or they simply can't be bothered. This aversion to exercise is borne out by data from the U.S. Centers for Disease Control (CDC) showing that in 2008, 36 percent of Americans reported no leisure time physical activity—a sad and frustrating state of affairs when doctors are continually telling their patients that they need to get active.

While the HHS report focuses on physical activity in a general sense, evidence also shows that running specifically confers some positive health benefits. Given that running is one of the simplest, most inexpensive, and accessible forms of aerobic exercise, this is good news. As an example, a 2008 study published in the *Archives of Internal Medicine* by Dr. Eliza Chakravarty of Stanford University and colleagues followed a group 538 runners and 423 healthy non-runners, all of age fifty or older, and found that after nineteen years, only 15 percent of runners had died, whereas 34 percent of non-running control subjects had died. Survival curves continued to diverge when data were looked at during the 21-year follow up—in other words, people who continue to run as they age have a decided survival advantage over non-runners. What's more, Dr. Chakrvarty's paper also shows that running reduces the incidence of disability later in life, so not only did the runners tend to live longer, they also tended to have a higher quality of life in their old age. Put simply, if you run, you'll have a higher chance of living a longer life, and you'll be more likely to be healthy in your old age than someone who does not run. Once again, it's hard to argue that these benefits aren't worth any risk or hardship that might be associated with running. "Running—it reduces your chance of dying!" is a mighty powerful message.

What Causes Runners to Get Hurt?

Given all of the positive health benefits associated with running, there are major incentives for both new and long-time runners to keep at it. Unfortunately, one thing that complicates matters when it comes to running and health is the fact that many runners get hurt. Indeed, a 2007 review by R. N. van Gent and colleagues in the *British Journal of Sports Medicine* (BJSM) looked at seventeen past studies on running injuries and indicated that the overall incidence of injury reported ranged from 19.4 to 79.3 percent. Those odds of getting hurt don't instill much confidence if one is looking to take up running as a way to get healthy. Must someone endure pain and suffering to reduce his or her chance of premature death? Are there ways a runner can reduce injury risk?

The question of why runners get injured is a difficult one to answer, and it's a question that has challenged health care practitioners, scientists, and runners alike for many years. A number of scientific studies have attempted to address this question by surveying runners and correlating various factors—training, gear, lifestyle and physical traits, biomechanical factors—with injury type suffered. For example, a 1992 article in the journal *Sports Science* by Willem van Mechelen of the University of Amsterdam analyzed existing literature on running injuries and found that only the following *four* factors could be clearly implicated as potential causes of running injury: previous injury, lack of running experience (see "New Runners At Risk"), running to compete, and excessive weekly running distance. Based on these findings, if you are a new runner with a history of knee problems who picks up the sport with a goal of completing a marathon within six months, you're pretty much doomed. Few would likely disagree with this prognosis.

New Runners at Risk

One of the most vulnerable times for a runner in terms of injury risk is when they are first starting out. Indeed, a 2010 study headed by Ida Buist of the University of Groningen and published in the *British Journal of Sports Medicine* looked at risk factors predisposing recreational runners to injury while training for a 4-mile race. Of particular interest is that this study included a large number of new runners, as well as a large number of runners who were just getting back into running after a period of time with no running. What was the report's conclusion? The strongest association found was that new runners are more likely to get injured than experienced runners, and that many of these runners, once injured, stopped running altogether.

What explains the risk faced by new runners? First of all, new runners are least adapted to the stresses and strains associated with running. Until strengthening and physical adaptation occur, injury risk is high. Second, lack of running experience limits their ability to distinguish minor aches from more serious pains—more experienced runners tend to have a better sense when a pain is abnormal and should be listened to. "Listen to your body" is an oft-repeated mantra among runners when it comes to knowing when to ease off, and new runners are far less fluent in the language of the running body. Third, determination to accomplish a pre-set goal (for example, finishing one's first marathon) might cause a new and inexperienced runner to push through clearly evident warning signs. All of these things set the stage for a an injury to occur, and a runner who is just starting out would be perhaps most wise to take things slow and gradual. It's for this reason alone that many coaches and sports doctors suggest holding off on attempting a marathon until one has been running for at least a year or two—this helps the body to adjust over time to the stresses of training for such a physically and mentally demanding event.

More recent injury association studies haven't been much more revealing. For example, the previously mentioned 2007 *BJSM* injury review by van Gent concluded that the following associations were the only ones that were *strongly* supported by existing injury data:

1. Altering training by increasing weekly training distance was reported to be protective against knee injuries. Wait, more mileage was better? Yes, this somewhat surprising finding was supported by two separate studies that the authors of the review had classified as "high-quality."
2. Training for more than sixty-four kilometers (forty miles) in a week was a significant risk factor for lower extremity injuries in males, but such an association was found in only one high-quality study for females.
3. No association was found between the use of a warm-up and lower extremity injury.
4. No association was found in males between injury incidence and running surface, hilly terrain, or running in the dark or in the morning.
5. History of previous injury was found to be a significant risk factor in multiple studies and for both sexes—this was one of the most significant factors found.

In the discussion of their results, van Gent's review points out the complex and sometimes contradictory findings reported in injury studies. For example, it reports that several studies found older age to be a risk factor for injury, but these were contradicted by others that found older age to be protective—conflicting evidence like this obviously makes firm conclusions difficult. Some of the results were also quite perplexing—for example, a 1999 study in the *British Journal of Sports Medicine* by Peter Satterthwaite and colleagues reported that drinking alcohol was a risk factor for developing blisters while running, whereas smoking was protective against blistering. This finding suggests that if you head out for a beer the night before a marathon, you should also smoke a cigarette so that you cancel out your risk! In all seriousness, even the authors of that study admit that it's "difficult to suggest a plausible explanation" for any direct link between drinking, smoking, and blistering.

Another interesting finding reported by van Gent was that body weight is not a strong predictor of running injury risk. In fact, a 1998 study by Dennis Wen and colleagues in the *Clinical Journal of Sports*

Medicine found that greater body weight was protective against foot injuries, and a study by Jack Taunton and colleagues in a 2003 issue of the *British Journal of Sports Medicine* found that a body mass index of 26 kg/m^2 or higher actually reduced the risk for male runners of suffering a lower extremity injuries. The notion that increased body weight might be protective against injuries seems to fly in the face of common sense, and the authors speculate that these counterintuitive results could stem from the fact that heavier runners might run fewer miles (probably at a slower pace). Such is the complexity of teasing apart multiple interacting factors in order to try to figure out why runners might be getting hurt—a lot of speculation and guesswork are involved.

Sadly, short of a few obvious factors (being a new runner, logging big miles, having a previous injury, being competitive), existing data on factors that increase or decrease risk of running injury are largely inconclusive, and can point to very little with any degree of certainty. The specific causes of running injury remain elusive, and too many runners are left to muddle along trying to figure out why it is that they get hurt.

Groups vs. Individuals: The Limitations of Running Injury Studies

Scientific studies have helped to identify some of the major factors that increase injury risk among runners, but it's important to recognize that injury association studies like those discussed in this chapter also have limitations. First, the conclusions that these studies make are typically based on statistical analyses of masses of data collected from a specific group. Thus, they report whether given factors are significantly associated with injury for the population of runners that was studied. As a result, the characteristics of the population being studied play a significant role in what the results might look like and how they should be interpreted. For example, perhaps a study looked at injuries among a group of experienced marathon runners with a mean age of thirty, and you are a fifty-year-old runner just starting out with a goal of completing a 5 kilometer race. In other words, you don't fit the demographics of study population, and thus it can be difficult to know if the results of the study are applicable to you.

It's also important to remember that just because a factor seems to increase injury likelihood in a sample of runners does not mean that it resulted in an injury in every individual in that sample. Human variability is the norm rather than the exception, and what applies to most may not apply to all. For example, the fact that high mileage training has been associated with a greater chance of injury does not mean that the moment you run more than 40 miles in a week your knee is going to pop. Statistical analyses are very good at inferring majority trends and associations, but they are not necessarily going to be 100 percent accurate when considering the individual. Some individuals might run 40 or more mile weeks repeatedly without a problem; others might run only 10-mile weeks and develop an injury. The statistics simply say that your chance of injury rises if you exceed the 40 mile threshold, not that you will get injured when you do.

Because of their strong reliance on statistical relationships and majority patterns, academic studies also have limitations when it comes to applicability in a clinical setting. Clinicians work with individual patients, not groups. A clinician is generally concerned with treating the individual who is sitting in front of them, and what might be best for that individual might not be best for all humans, or even a majority. Thus, although academic studies can provide excellent guidance regarding therapeutic approaches that might work in a given situation, health care practitioners also utilize their own clinical experience when devising treatment strategies. For example, a physical therapist likely has developed a body of knowledge through years of practice regarding which treatments typically work best for a given injury. These treatments may or may not be supported by academic research, but the fact that a study does not exist to support a particular approach should not preclude them from using it if they have employed it with outstanding success in the past.

Types of Running Injuries—A "Walk" Through Time

Ah, the good old days of running. Runners hear that line a lot, usually from those who started running in the 1960s and 1970s. Was there really a golden age of running when runners seldom came up lame from an injury? Or is this a mere fiction, an invention or reordering of memory? By the same token, there's that uncomfortable feeling that running injuries are a modern problem, a byproduct of cushioned shoes with lifted heels, and that runners in the stripped-down shoes of the earlier era were somehow immune from injuries. Unfortunately, the truth is not quite that simple.

In his 1935 book "*Running*," Arthur Newton includes an entire chapter titled "Troubles." In the chapter's opening paragraph, Newton writes that injury is no stranger to runners:

> *{Real} intensive training can produce an amazing crop, at any rate during the early stages. If you have nothing else to brag about you can admire the heterogeneous assortment of brand new and unexpected "aggranoyances" it showers promiscuously around. To hint at only a few . . . blisters, cramp, stitch, colds, uneasy joints, and sinews together with their accompanying holocaust of invigorated language . . .*

Newton had more than a casual familiarity with running injuries. He'd occasionally log well over 200 miles of running per week on rough South African roads while in his forties—this type of mileage is likely to cause problems for anyone. Furthermore, despite his own masochistic mileage totals, he believed that running was less likely to cause injury compared to other athletic pursuits if "you indulge in moderation only." As a perceptive student of human behavior, Newton also addressed how to manage injuries, humorously reporting that there are "remedies which sportsmen have employed all along and which certainly work wonders . . . (a) grouse, and (b) persistence in regarding them as a joke."

Running injuries are nothing new, which means that the shoe company giants can hardly be ascribed sole blame for the current plague of running woes. However, detailed accounts of injuries are difficult to come by prior to the 1970s. It wasn't until the early 1970s that a more systematic documentation of running injuries became commonplace, and much of this early work came in the form of injury surveys conducted by a relatively new magazine (at the time) called *Runner's World*.

In 1980, highly respected running biomechanist Peter Cavanagh (currently the endowed chair of Women's Sports Medicine at the University of Washington) wrote a book titled *The Running Shoe Book*. In it, Cavanagh, who set up and directed the first shoe test lab for *Runner's World*, cited the 1971 results of the magazine's first reader survey of injuries. A total of 800 runners responded to the survey, and each reported the types of "major" foot and leg injuries they had sustained—"major" was defined as "requiring a complete layoff from running." The five most common injuries reported were:

1. Knee injury (17.9%)
2. Achilles tendon injury (14%)
3. Shin splints (10.6%)
4. Arch injury (6.9%)
5. Ankle injury (6.4%)

Runner's World's survey was conducted again in 1973; 1,680 runners reported a total of 1,600 injuries (some runners reported more than one). The top five injuries were:

1. Knee injury (22.5%)
2. Achilles tendon injury (20.3%)
3. Shin splints (9.9%)
4. Forefoot injury (7.2%)
5. Heel injury (7.2%)

Cavanagh highlighted that "the shoes used by runners in the 1971–1973 period were lacking in what we now believe to be important protective characteristics," and that shoes from this period "were heavy, thin under the forepart, lacking in shock absorption, and provided a relatively small differential in height between the heel and forefoot." As an example of such a shoe, Cavanagh reports that the second most popular shoe in 1971 was the Adidas Olympia, which weighed over 12 ounces and had a gum-rubber sole with no midsole or heel wedge.

Cavanagh went on to cite 1979 injury statistics for 974 runners provided by the Runners Clinic of St. Elizabeth's Hospital in Massachusetts. The top five common injury types were:

1. Knee injury (30.5%),
2. Heel spur syndrome (includes plantar fasciitis; 13.5%),
3. Shin splints (10.9%),
4. Muscle pulls (8%), and
5. Achilles tendonitis (6%)

Cavanagh acknowledged the inherent limitations of the available data (for example, surveys vs. clinical data as well as injury terminology differences), but it was the best available data from that time period, and he made several interesting observations about how injury patterns changed from the early to late 1970s (a time when both running shoe design and runner demographics experienced dramatic changes). Cavanagh noted that within the span of ten years, Achilles tendon injuries, metatarsal stress fractures, ankle injuries, and heel bone injuries became less common, whereas knee injuries, shin splints (he combined shin splints and posterior tibial tendonitis percentages for 1979 since he felt that earlier surveys probably included both of these under the category "shin splints"), heel spur syndrome, and leg fractures (mostly tibial and fibular stress fractures) became considerably more common.

Even though knee injuries were the most common injury in each of these studies, Cavanagh was particularly concerned about the *rising* incidence of knee injuries in 1979. What caused this spike? He speculated that "the combination of poor skeletal alignment and high mileage is going to play its part in knee injuries," but also indicated that "we also have to examine the proposition, however unpalatable, that shoes, far from preventing injuries, have been partly responsible for them." How might this happen? Cavanagh felt that lifting and adding cushioning material under the heel might have helped alleviate Achilles tendon and heel injuries, but that a potential side effect of adding a heel wedge was "inferior rearfoot control." In other words, excessive pronation, the inward roll of the foot that occurs after ground contact, might have been the culprit that was increasingly damaging runner's knees as the decade progressed, and it might have been caused by the added elements in shoes that were put there in part to protect runners from Achilles tendon and foot problems.

In addition to alterations in shoe construction and the shift in frequencies of injury types, the profile of the average runner changed significantly during this period. By the end of the 1970s, running had become far more of a mainstream pastime. Amby Burfoot, editor-at-large for *Runner's World* and winner of the 1968 Boston Marathon, says that the "1970 runner was leaner, meaner and faster than the 1980 runner . . . virtually all (1970) runners were those who continued (running) from high school, college, military service. They were more talented and more closely connected to recent high-level fitness." In contrast, Burfoot points out that the average runner in 1980 was an individual "still in relative youth who picked up running after reading Jim Fixx's book, and began training hard. They might have put in a lot of miles, but many were inherently not that talented as runners when compared to the average runner of 1970." So the population of runners changed from mostly lifelong athletes to individuals who might have been joining the sport for the first time or who were returning to running later in life. Injury studies have shown that new runners are more likely to succumb to injury, so it's quite possible that this demographic shift contributed to the changing nature of running injuries over the course of the decade; but to what extent is difficult to estimate with any degree of certainty.

During the late 1970s and early 1980s, the development of running shoes went from being mostly an ad hoc or improvisational affair to one that was heavily influenced by emerging footwear science and research. "Running shoes came out of the dark age," wrote Cavanagh, and shoe design as it related to injury prevention became a topic of intense study by biomechanical researchers. One of the main concerns during this period was how to control excessive movement of the rearfoot, or what we now commonly refer to as "pronation control." The logic went like this: if the raised, cushioned heel of running shoes compromised rearfoot control, and this in turn contributed to the rising incidence of knee injuries, then something needed to be done to stabilize shoes and correct for this.

Thus began the "pronation-control paradigm" that would guide shoe design for years to come. Shoes now *required* structural elements whose intended purpose was to limit the amount of pronation that occurred after the foot made contact with the ground, most often on the outer portion of the heel. The hope was that by keeping excessive pronation in check, the number of knee injuries experienced by runners would be reduced. Over the next thirty years, devices like medial posts, dual density midsoles, flared heels, and rigid heel counters were introduced in a continuing attempt to control potentially harmful movements of the foot that may have been caused by the construction of the shoe itself (mainly their soft, compressible midsoles). These are the very same elements that are found in many modern running shoes; in fact, the level of pronation control continues to be the primary factor by which shoes are classified by manufacturers and in most stores today.

There is a lot more to say about the pronation-control paradigm, and we will cover it further in Chapter 6, but for now the most important question to address is this: what has been the effect of this added shoe technology on injuries? To attempt to answer this, let's review some of the injury studies discussed earlier.

Based on findings published in van Gent's 2007 review paper in the *British Journal of Sports Medicine,* as well as many others that have been published over the past three to four decades, it's clear that a lot of runners get injured every year, and that injury rates since 1980 have not diminished to any measureable extent. Furthermore, though injuries like shin splints, Achilles tendinopathy, ilitibial band syndrome and plantar fasciitis remain common, the knee continues to be the most frequently cited location of injury. All of these injuries continue despite immense, well-intentioned effort on the part of biomechanics experts and shoe companies to design shoes with characteristics aimed at preventing injury. Though much debate exists regarding the causes of the ongoing running injury epidemic, answers regarding why runners continue to get hurt at alarming rates remain as elusive as ever.

One possible contributing factor to the failure of scientific research and "improved" shoe technology to reduce injury rates is that runner demographics have changed perhaps even more dramatically in recent years than they did during the 1970's. Running is now more popular than ever as evidenced by the increased participation in distance running events from the 5K to the marathon (see "Today's Runner"). It is immediately apparent from watching runners cross the finish line at any race that runners come in all shapes and sizes. On average, runners today are probably significantly heavier in body weight and less physically fit than they were in 1980, and some suggest that this demographic change might explain why new shoe technology has failed to lower injury rates. In other words, the shoes are indeed better, but the runners are now worse.

Regarding the "good shoes, bad runner" hypothesis, it is important to point out that Body Mass Index (BMI) has not been consistently linked to increased risk of running injury. In fact, several studies have found no link between BMI and running injury risk, and as mentioned previously, some studies have found a higher BMI to actually be protective against injuries, perhaps since larger runners tend to run more slowly and log fewer miles. Furthermore, we doubt we are alone in knowing more than a few exceptionally fit, long-time runners who have succumbed to injury—the injury bug doesn't seem to single out only the unfit and overweight. Thus, the effects of demographic change in the running population on injury incidence are unclear at best.

Today's Runner

Over 500,000 runners finished a marathon in 2010, according to a published report by *Running USA*. The half-marathon number is even more staggering: 1.4 million finishers. Since 2003, the half-marathon has been the fastest growing road race distance in this country, with women making up 59 percent of the field. In the full marathon, men comprise 59 percent of the field.

The *Running USA* Half-Marathon Report offered the following reasons for the increase in half-marathon runners: "The popularity of the distance has been fueled mainly by charity and non-charity training programs, destination-type events/series, runners moving up or down from the marathon, and women's participation."

Because marathoners and half-marathoners are the ultimate number-crunchers, always thinking in terms of mile splits, minutes run per day, PRs, all the while logging training data into their favorite fitness apps, let's look at some other noteworthy statistics for 26.2 and 13.1.

- In 1897, the first Boston Marathon (just under 25 miles) debuted one year after the Athens Games with just fifteen starters. Ten runners finished. By 1902, the field swelled to forty-two runners, with over 100,000 spectators lining the course.
- It wasn't until 1964 that more than 300 runners entered the Boston Marathon.
- In 1976, 25,000 runners finished a marathon in the U.S.
- The average age of a male marathon finisher today is forty; for women it's thirty-six.
- The average finishing time of a male marathoner today is 4:27; for women it's 4:54.
- The top seven marathons in the U.S. based on the total number of 2010 finishers: New York City (44,704); Chicago (36,159), Boston (22,540), Los Angeles (22,403); Marine Corps (21,974); Honolulu (20,169); Disney World (16,874).
- In 2010, there were 664 official marathon finishes in the U.S. under 2:30, and more than 9,000 finishes under 3:00.
- The number of masters (age forty and older) who finished a marathon in 1980 in the U.S. was 10 percent; by 2010, the number increased to 46 percent.

- The number of juniors (under twenty years old) who finished a marathon in 1980 in the U.S. was 5 percent; by 2010, the number decreased to 2 percent.
- Of the largest timed road race events in the United States, 42 percent of them are half-marathons.
- Since 1995, the number of female finishers in the half-marathon has increased by a factor of six (135,000 women in 1995 to 820,000 in 2010).
- Seven of the top fifteen women-only events in the nation are half-marathons.
- Average age of a half-marathon finisher: men (thirty-nine); women (thirty-six).
- Average time of a half-marathon finisher: men (2:00); women (2:19).

Repetitive Stress and Running Injury

Given the significant positive health benefits conferred by running, the lack of concrete information on what causes runners to get hurt, and the complexity of interpreting the information that is available, what should a runner who simply wants to run pain and injury free for better health do? Our intent here is not to provide a detailed recounting of every possible running injury that you might suffer and how you might best avoid them. Rather, let's consider the primary underlying factor at the core of nearly every one of the injuries mentioned in this chapter: repetitive stress. Combine the repetitive stress of running with an ill-fitting pair of shoes or poor running mechanics (or both) and high running mileage, and a nagging pain somewhere in the lower extremities is a not infrequent result. Add in a bit of fatigue and some stubbornly obsessive determination that causes you to ignore internal warning signs, and you have the makings of a full-blown disaster!

There's no escaping the obvious: running can be hard on the human body. With every running step you impact the ground with a force equivalent to approximately 2 to 3 times your body weight. Your joints compress, your muscles stretch and contract, and your tendons and ligaments tug and rub on bones. On average, you take some 80 to 95 running steps per minute with each foot. Extrapolate that over a thirty-minute run and you are dealing with 2400 to 2850 impacts per foot, per half-hour—that's a lot of stress for the body to take. Fortunately, your muscles, tendons, ligaments, bones, and joint surfaces are usually up to the task and do an excellent job of absorbing this repetitive shock. Furthermore, some degree of stress is actually essential to keeping the body's tissues healthy and strong. Think about what happens when you immobilize a broken limb in a cast—it gets weak, and strengthening exercise is necessary to restore the limb to its pre-injury state when the cast is removed. Staying active keeps body tissues healthy, and prolonged inactivity generally contributes to a decline in overall health.

As an example of the fact that physical stress is not always such a bad thing, let's consider briefly the runner's knee. Despite the common belief among non-runners that distance runners ruin their knees when pounding the pavement, a 2008 study on knee osteoarthritis headed by Dr. Eliza Chakravarty from Stanford University (the same doctor who wrote the article on reduced death rates among aging runners discussed earlier) showed that runner's knees are no worse off over the long term than those of non-runners, and there was even a trend showing that knee osteoarthritis was actually less prevalent among runners (20% in runners vs. 32% in non-runners). Although the difference was not statistically significant, the trend indicates that some level of stress on the knee from running may actually be protective against osteoarthritis. Chakravarty expressed surprise in an interview with health and fitness writer Gretchen Reynolds of the *New York Times,* stating that "Our hypothesis going in had been that runners, because of the repetitive pounding, would develop more frequent and more severe arthritis." Their results revealed that this was clearly not the case. So, the next time someone tells you that your knees are being wrecked by running, you can simply share with your antagonist the findings from Dr. Chakravarty's articles. Your running knees might actually be better off, and there's a decent chance you might live longer and with better quality of life in your old age.

Why Runners Get Hurt

Although physical stress is important for keeping the body strong, stress cannot be applied indefinitely. Stress the body too much without allowing time for rest and repair, and eventually it will break down, particularly if the stress is being applied in a new way that the body is not used to. This is the fundamental process by which most running injuries develop.

Injuries incurred as a result of running can be classified into two major groupings. First there are acute injuries. These are injuries that happen suddenly, usually resulting from some form of traumatic event. You might be running down a mountain trail a bit too quickly, trip over a rock or root, and sprain your ankle or mash up your knee. You might collide with a sign-pole or tree while running in the dark (don't laugh, this has happened to both coauthors). The point here is that an acute injury is usually the result of some form of accident—it happens all-of-a-sudden and you can usually pinpoint the cause. The other type of injuries are more common among runners; these are repetitive stress or overuse injuries. As the name implies, repetitive stress injuries result from activities that repeatedly tax the body in a similar manner. The individual stresses that lead to such an injury may in fact be quite small, but because they are repeated over and over again their cumulative effects can be quite large, which can trigger an injury. Because this type of injury generally develops over an extended period of time, it can often be quite difficult to pinpoint its exact cause.

Runners are especially susceptible to repetitive stress injuries because running is a highly repetitive behavior. Even if everything else is perfect (for example, no underlying biomechanical or anatomical problems), this level of repetitive stress alone can be problematic if the body is not adapted to it—hence why new runners often suffer from aches and pains shortly after starting a running program (see "New Runners at Risk"). However, if some aspect of your gait is flawed, repetitive stress can be amplified and the likelihood of developing a problem increases. Let's take iliotibial band syndrome (ITBS) as an example. The iliotibial band (ITB) is a strap of connective tissue that originates from the hip, extends down the side of the thigh, and attaches to both the femur (thigh bone) and tibia (shin bone) on the outer side of the knee. Suppose a muscular imbalance in the hips caused the thigh on one side to angle inward (adduction) to a greater degree than it should as it swings forward in preparation for landing. As a result, the foot might cross the midline when it strikes the ground. This, in turn, could place excessive tension on the ITB, and could cause a greater amount of friction between the ITB and the bone underlying it. Over the course of a few strides this might not pose much of a problem, but do it several thousand times in rapid succession and it's no surprise that you might start feeling a bit of discomfort on the outer side of your knee joint. Such is the nature of repetitive stress (see "Muscle Imbalances and the Modern Runner").

Muscle Imbalances and the Modern Runner

In an ideal world all of your muscles would function in complete harmony while you run. Each muscle would do its job while in just the right position and with just the right amount of force applied at just the right time to allow you to move fluidly and painlessly over the ground below. Unfortunately, our bodies are rarely perfect. You break down your tissues via everyday wear and tear, you accommodate for aches and pains by changing your gait and shifting loads to uninjured tissues, and some of your muscles tend to work harder than others. All of these things can lead to the development of muscle imbalances and asymmetries. These imbalances, in turn, can cause gait abnormalities that have the potential to precipitate injuries.

For one example, right-left imbalances in muscle strength/function are common. Seemingly benign behaviors like driving a car on a daily commute (you work the gas pedal and brake with the right foot while the left foot does nothing), running on the same side of a cambered road, or always carrying a baby/toddler on the same hip can lead to the development of imbalances in muscle strength between the two sides of the body. Imbalances created by asymmetrical behaviors like these can have significant impact on your ability to properly control your body when you run. For example, right-left imbalances in hip abductor (gluteus medius) strength have been linked to such common injuries as iliotibial band syndrome and patellofemoral pain syndrome.

Jay Dicharry, a physical therapist at the University of Virginia, and head of the SPEED Lab at the UVA Center for Endurance Sport, emphasizes that that imbalances such as these are not inherent problems with the human body, but rather stem from how most people use their bodies on an everyday basis. "If you think about how our body was designed, it was designed very well," says Dicharry, "It's what our society has done to our body that changes our soft tissue structure." How do you know if you have an imbalance that might be contributing to an ache or pain? Best to see a health expert like Dicharry—a trained medical professional well versed in the structure and function of the human body who can help you track down the source of your problems and develop a plan for putting your body back into balance.

The repetitive-stress problem is exacerbated by the fact that many runners run most of their miles on uniform, hard surfaces—roads, sidewalks and the like. And they do this day in, day out. However, it may not be the hardness of these modern surfaces that causes problems (more on this in the next chapter), rather it might be the uniformity of one's training and running surfaces that is the bigger issue. Many runners run repeatedly on roads and sidewalks near their homes, often on the same routes over and over, and there is very little variation in a concrete or asphalt surface. Running on unvarying asphalt forces the joints to flex, extend, compress, and decompress in nearly the exact same way with every step, concentrating stress on a few specific parts of the lower extremity. However, when you decide to change things up and move to a trail, your feet and legs are constantly adapting to variations in the ground surface, and they get worked more thoroughly than when running on a road. Running on a trail with an irregular surface is very different, and it doesn't take long for a road runner to start feeling leg fatigue when they decide to hit the trail—muscles that are not often used during road running get called into action and are not ready for the added variety and stabilization work that running on irregular trails requires. Trail running likely increases risk of acute injuries from tripping on roots or rocks, but the variety in surface underfoot may protect against repetitive overuse injury to some degree.

The point of this brief discussion of surface is that the more repetitive your running is, and the more often you run repetitively, the greater the likelihood that you will suffer a repetitive overuse injury by stressing the same spot over and over. This risk, in turn, may be exacerbated and amplified by such things as form flaws, footwear problems, muscle imbalances, or anatomical abnormalities. As an example of how some of these factors can mesh together to cause an injury, let's focus on stress fractures of bones.

The Adaptable Human Body

A common misperception held by many people (including many of Pete's students in his Human Anatomy class) is that bones are nothing more than hard white things inside your flesh that help to hold the body together and prevent you from collapsing into a pile of mush on the floor. While bones do in fact do these things, they are actually dynamic, adaptable structures that are considerably more complex in their structure and function than most typically give them credit for.

Your bones are quite remarkable in that they are capable of going through a process known as remodeling. What this means essentially is that your bones can change shape to better withstand the forces that you habitually expose them to. You have cells in and on your bones called osteoclasts and osteoblasts that can break down old and build up new bone, and they do a very good job of it. When you stress a particular spot on a bone repeatedly, it begins to develop micro-damage—think of micro-damage as tiny cracks that weaken a bone in that spot. The remodeling process repairs that damage, and ultimately will make the bone stronger and better able to withstand that stress. The catch is that remodeling takes time, and the damaged spot actually gets a bit weaker (as damaged bone is removed by osteoclast cells) before it is repaired and becomes stronger. If you repeatedly stress a bone in the same way over and over without giving it a chance to rest and repair, micro-damage accumulates and can lead to a stress fracture. If you continue to stress a bone that has already developed a stress fracture, you can imagine what will happen next—snap!

This same type of process applies to many soft tissue injuries as well, and muscles are a good example. When you go lift weights for the first time in a long time you get incredibly sore for the next few days (this is called delayed onset muscle soreness or DOMS). What has happened is that you have damaged your muscles on a microscopic level, and as they repair themselves they become larger and stronger. This is the fundamental process by which you are able to increase strength through resistance training. However, if you decide to start working out and you do the same routine every day for a week or two, you're asking for trouble. One can apply this same logic to an extent to cartilage, ligaments, and tendons as well, though they typically have a harder time repairing themselves due to their more limited blood supply. The body is amazingly good at adapting, you just need to allow it time to do so.

As discussed previously, overuse injuries occur when repeated stresses are placed upon a structure, none of which individually causes acute damage, but the sum of which leads to a progressive degeneration of that structure. In simple terms, if you pound on a bone too frequently without rest, it's eventually going to break. If you overstretch or apply excessive friction to a ligament repeatedly, it's eventually going to get sore and possibly tear. You get the picture. A helpful way to think of this is demonstrated by the graph below, adapted from a 2004 article by Alan Hreljac in the journal *Medicine and Science in Sport and Exercise*.

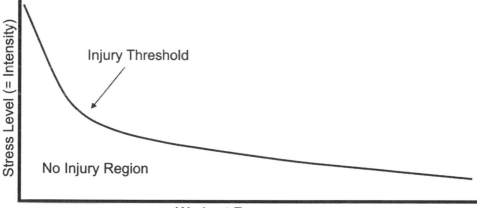

The above graph looks at training and injury likelihood as a balance of intensity and frequency. High intensity workouts (for example, hard speedwork, long runs) are more taxing on the body and would score high on the "stress level" axis. Thus, if they are done frequently your training will exceed the injury threshold (the curved black line) and you're asking for a problem. However, if your workout is low intensity (a short recovery run at a slow pace), you can do that workout frequently and not likely get hurt (you will remain in the "no injury" region below the curve).

The thing to keep in mind in the above graph is that the exact shape and height of the curve will likely vary from person to person (some people are simply more injury prone than others, some can tolerate hard workouts better than others), from time to time within a single individual (with degree of overall fatigue, how recently one has started running), perhaps with sudden change to a different running surface (treadmill vs. irregular dirt trail vs. asphalt/concrete), and even in different pairs of shoes. As an example of the latter, when a person used to wearing heavily cushioned shoes with a prominent heel lift goes for their first run in a pair of ultraminimal, barefoot-style shoes which lack a heel lift and are minimally cushioned, the entire injury threshold curve probably shifts downward (see dashed line in graph on following page). Thus, in runners just starting out in ultraminimal shoes, even low intensity runs should not be done frequently at the start, and high intensity runs can cause problems immediately. Most importantly, you don't want your first run in an ultraminimal shoe to be an all out 5K race or a 20 mile marathon training run).

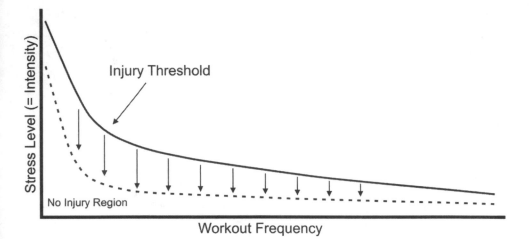

After the first run in an ultraminimal shoe is complete, delayed onset soreness in places like the calf muscles is a common outcome. This likely lowers the injury threshold even further prior to the next run, and this is why running too much too soon (TMTS) is to be avoided at all costs when adapting to a barefoot-style shoe like the Vibram FiveFingers or any other ultraminimal shoe. Adapting to barefoot-style shoes requires a very low-intensity initial approach with a very gradual build-up—to do otherwise dramatically increases your likelihood of injury. The metatarsal bones in your foot and the muscles, tendons, and ligaments of the feet and legs need time to adapt to the new forces that they are experiencing when running in these shoes. As the adaptation process proceeds, the bones and muscles get stronger, and the dashed line will start to rise back upward, and along with it the risk of injury should decline (the rate and degree to which this occurs is likely to be individually variable).

Several factors are critical to helping a runner minimize the risk of suffering an overuse injury such as a stress fracture, and the first is to take a gradual approach to any kind of change and allow for plenty of rest. If you begin exposing bones to a new form of stress, such as greater force applied to the metatarsal heads or increased bending torques on the metatarsal shafts when you start running barefoot or in a barefoot-style shoe, you need to allow the bones time to remodel to better withstand these new stresses. This is particularly important if you adopt a forefoot strike, and even more so if you try to run up on your toes and not let the heel come down after initial contact on the forefoot is made—a rapid transition to a forced/exaggerated forefoot strike can put tremendous stress on delicate foot bones that are not accustomed to this type of force application. Strengthening the feet takes time, just like strengthening any other part of the body—patience is required, and attempting to force change in an exaggerated manner is a big mistake.

Failure to exercise caution by following a very gradual adaptation approach is likely a significant contributing factor to the occurrence of metatarsal stress fractures and other types of overuse injuries in new barefoot and/or barefoot-style runners. In fact, "too much too soon" or "TMTS" is often suggested (and self-reported) as the causative agent among new barefoot-style runners who develop repetitive overuse injuries during the transition period. Runners get overly exuberant about trying a new thing that they read about in a book, on a blog, or in the newspaper, buy a pair of barefoot-style/ultraminimalist shoes, and run every day for a week in them at their normal training mileage. It's a recipe for disaster, and the result is that their bodies rapidly start to break down.

The logic behind adapting gradually to barefoot-style footwear can be equally applied to many other types of changes that might occur in your training. For example, if you were to go out and run a hard interval session every day for a week after not doing speedwork for several months, your chance of suffering an injury is likely quite high. If your body is not used to the stress you expose it to, whether it be from a new shoe or a new type of workout, the chances are good that it will suffer in some way. If, however, you start out slow, build gradually, and allow plenty of rest, you provide a dose of the new stress that the body can manage. Then, the body adapts to better withstand new stresses on future runs, and breakdowns are less likely. Rest is critical to this process, and failure to do so may guarantee you a trip the doctor's office.

In addition to allowing time for rest and repair, a potentially effective approach to avoiding repetitive overuse injury is to simply break the cycle of repetitive stress by adding variability to your workouts. This can be accomplished in a number of ways. For example, rather than running all of your miles in the same shoes over the same route on the same roads around your home, change things up and run on trails from time to time. Your gait changes as you run on different surfaces, and changes in joint angles can alter how force is applied to the limbs. This, in turn, can help you avoid constantly straining your feet and legs in the same way on every run. In a similar manner, doing something as simple as not always running on the same side of the road can be of benefit (as long as it can be done safely). Most roads are cambered, meaning that they are highest in the middle and slope downward to each side to facilitate water runoff. The problem with this for a runner is that when running on the side of the road, one foot is usually landing slightly higher than the other due to the slope. If this is never varied by running on the opposite side of the road from time to time, it can lead to imbalances and other problems that might ultimately trigger an injury. Varying speed can also be of benefit— as with surface, your gait changes with speed, and mixing up your pace from time to time might help reduce the repetitive stress load.

Another way to break the cycle of repetitive stress that some runners find to be of benefit is to rotate among several pairs of shoes. The logic to this approach is that each shoe will stress the body in a slightly different way given its structural makeup (things like heel height, cushioning thickness, sole firmness, arch support), and thus rotating a few pairs of shoes might help vary the specific locations of force application in the lower limbs. There is not any hard data to support this approach, and rotating too many shoes could actually be detrimental since it prevents adaptation to any one pair, but it seems reasonable to assume that by moving stress points around as one varies footwear, the legs and feet will become stronger and more injury resistant all around.

Thou Shalt Not Run a Marathon in a New Pair of Shoes

In late 2010, I broke one of the most sacred of running commandments— Thou Shalt Not Run a Marathon in a New Pair of Shoes. I had received a new pair of racing flats to review for my website *Runblogger*, and after a single solid but fatiguing long run in them I decided I was going to wear them in the Manchester City (NH) Marathon one week later. I had intended for this race to be more of a "fun" run since I knew I would be fatigued after having run a Boston qualifying effort in the Smuttynose Rockfest Marathon only a month earlier. I had agreed to help a friend pace the 3:40 finishing group, and given that this would be a considerably slower pace than I had run in my previous race, the prospect of running in a shiny new pair of shoes was rather intriguing—what could possibly go wrong? There were, however, several big problems with my logic. First, I had never run a marathon in true road racing flats. Second, the shoes were new and my feet and legs had not had time to adjust to them. Third, I was fatigued, and a marathon is a very, very long race.

I decided to throw caution to the wind and wear the flats on race day. I started feeling sore in both my feet and legs early in the race, particularly on the left side, and as a result I ignored any attempt to pay attention to my form—I opted to just let my body find the way to run that hurt the least. I think the soreness led to some odd gait alteration on the left side, and by late race, around mile 20, my left iliotibial band and hip flexor were both barking at me loudly. I finished the race just under the target time (mission accomplished, despite the pain!), but dealt with some residual soreness under the outside of my left foot over the week following the race.

Although residual fatigue and a hilly course were surely factors that contributed to my troubles, the shoes I wore for the race gave me similar problems on subsequent runs so they clearly played a role as well. I've since determined that they simply weren't a good fit for me, and because I hadn't trained much in them prior to the race, I didn't know that ahead of time. This is why getting familiar with shoes before running an intense effort in them is always a smart approach.

I took my customary break from running for several days after the marathon to allow some time for my body to recover and repair, and though pain in my foot had subsided, I was still aware that things were not quite right. Nonetheless, my need to run got the better of me, so I decided to test things out on an easy recovery run. About halfway into the run, the pain in my left foot flared up to the point where I had stop running. I was forced to hobble my way home. I was worried that I had done some real damage. Panic was beginning to set in.

Through a combination of my knowing a thing or two about anatomy and a little Google medical sleuthing (not advocating this approach, just being honest!), I determined that the problem seemed to be some inflammation in one of my peroneal tendons that extended under the outside of my left ankle to the underside of my foot. I was left with a few options. One would be to avoid running for awhile longer and see if the injury resolved itself. The second would be to see a medical professional and get it checked out (probably the wise option). Third would be to employ a shoe rotation technique that I had used many times previously with positive results. The method works like this: when a bout of unusual soreness pops up on a run,

I've found that by choosing a shoe on subsequent runs that has a slightly different structural makeup, I can continue running and the pain eventually goes away. What I think happens is that I rest the strained spot by using a shoe that alters force application and/or muscle activation in some way and thus concentrates stresses and strains in a slightly different area—this is probably not dissimilar to how orthotics work.

I opted for option number three, and decided that I would attempt my next run in a pair of shoes with a more substantial heel lift (9mm heel-forefoot height differential compared to the 4mm differential of the flats)—this was only two days after hobbling home in pain. The vast majority of my runs are in shoes with a differential of 6mm or less, so this shoe was structurally a lot different than what I'm used to. Thus, my hope was that it would alter the stress application on my foot in a way that might allow me to run without pain.

I left the house tentatively, planning to cut the run short at the slightest twinge of discomfort. It never came. I picked up the pace, and the foot still felt good. I was still aware that there was something "off" in my left foot, but it never hurt during the run, and I couldn't have been happier. The pain resolved in fairly short order, and I was able to go back to my preferred shoe style with no recurring issues.

The point of this story is that making a sudden change to your training, whether it be in distance, intensity, or type of shoe worn, can increase your likelihood of suffering an injury. Running a tough, long race on only a month's rest is clearly the ultimate reason why I got hurt—if I skipped the race, chances are I would not have had any problems. But, running the race in a shoe that I was not used to and that turned out to be a poor match for me amplified my risk. Based on this experience and others I've become a firm believer that the wrong pair of shoes can cause an injury. At the same time, my experience also demonstrates that sometimes making a change in footwear to something slightly (or even substantially) different is all it takes to alter stresses in such a way that a nagging pain can be alleviated. It may not always work, but it has worked for me on more than one occasion. Perhaps most importantly, the entire incident has taught me that injuries are often multifactorial in their cause—mix together the wrong combination of distance, intensity, and footwear and problems can crop up that might not have otherwise happened.   —PML

Summary

Repetitive stress, and a failure to allow the body time to adapt to it, is the primary cause of running injuries. Poor training decisions (often translated to mean overtraining and spending insufficient time for rest and recovery) are why most runners exceed their individual repetitive stress threshold—in other words, runners tend to run too hard or too long, and do so too often for their individual levels of fitness and physical adaptation. To reduce the likelihood of an overuse injury (and all the baggage that comes with it), it's wise to take a sensible approach to training as well as racing. Whenever possible, attempt to break the cycle of repetitive stress, rest when needed, and be wary of making any change (for example, new shoes or training methods) too quickly.

With that said, runners tend to be a stubborn and persistent lot. Even if a runner is suffering a persistent ache somewhere below the waist, the need to get a run in can often outweigh the potential that the ache might turn into something worse. So listen to your body. Try not to ignore what it's saying.

CHAPTER 3

✺

Barefoot and Running

*I found [shoes] uncomfortable and after that I decided to con-
tinue running barefoot because I found it more comfortable. I
felt more in touch with what was happening. I could actually
feel the track.*

—Zola Budd

It's clearly a paradox: humans are exceptionally good at running long
distances, but when modern runners do so with regularity they have an
exceedingly high tendency to get hurt. The propensity for distance running to cause repetitive stress injuries makes little sense or logic from an
evolutionary perspective—our ancestors wouldn't have been able to run
down dinner if they were constantly sidelined by overuse injuries. Unfortunately, we'll never know how frequently *Homo erectus* or early *Homo
sapiens* might have been struck down by a bad case of Achilles tendinopathy or plantar fasciitis, so it's difficult to assess whether modern injury
rates for runners are an aberration. However, if the persistence hunting
hypothesis is correct and distance running was critical to the ability of
our ancestors to obtain food, then it seems unlikely that repetitive stress
injuries could have been as common as they are now.

One thing we do know though is that a lot has changed over the past
two million years. Running in the modern, developed world is in many
ways quite different from that practiced by our ancestors. Today's runners
wear technical polyester fabrics rather than animal skins; they consume
energy bars, gels and sports drinks instead of meats, roots, vegetables and
fruits; they log miles for fun or out of a desire to compete, often by fol-

lowing detailed workout plans, instead of out of necessity for survival; they run for the most part on concrete and asphalt instead of rock, sand, and dirt; and they are almost always shod in cushioned shoes rather than running in their bare feet.

In this chapter we turn our attention to the topic of barefoot running. The aim is not to convince you to empty your closet of all of your running shoes. Instead, we hope to take a balanced look at the barefoot-running debate, and shed further light on the complex relationship between the human foot and the running shoe.

Barefoot Running: Past and Present

Humans clearly evolved to run barefoot, of that there is little doubt. Our running ancestors honed their endurance skills with unshod feet, much like every other running animal on this planet. However, as the human species evolved, it entered into new habitats where the environmental conditions were vastly different, and often quite a bit colder, than those in Africa where man first originated. For example, it's rather unlikely that humans inhabiting ice age Europe were trotting around with regularity in their bare feet. One of the adaptations that humans possess as a species is the ability to use their intelligence and resourcefulness to invent devices that might help them to survive in those new habitats, and shoes are an effective means of protecting the feet from cold or rough ground underfoot.

Although going barefoot was the norm for *Homo erectus* several million years ago, a simple glance at the feet of runners at the starting line of most any modern-day race makes it clear that running shoe companies need have no fear that barefoot runners will lead a mass movement away from shoes. The shoe-buying public is here to stay. The athletic footwear industry alone is a multi-billion dollar colossus.

Few people in the developed world are running barefoot full-time. The reasons are many—for some, it's simple practicality. Whether it be unsuitably cold winter weather, or a lack of suitable barefoot running surfaces, there are certain situations in which running barefoot is simply not possible. For others it may be self-consciousness—the thought of trotting around barefoot is just too much of a social abnormality for them to imagine doing it. Whatever the reasons, full-time barefoot running will never become the norm in this day and age. However, important lessons can be learned from those who do run in their bare feet, and in recent years the number of individuals running barefoot with regularity has been growing.

Despite all the media-fueled excitement surrounding barefoot running, it is by no means a new practice, even in more recent history. For example, some runners have competed barefoot at the highest level—Olympians Abebe Bikila of Ethiopia and Zola Budd of South Africa (Budd competed for Great Britain in the 1984 Los Angeles Olympics) come immediately to mind. Barefoot strides on grass have long been employed by track and cross country runners as a method for improving form, as well as for strengthening the legs and feet. Some well-known coaches have even recommended barefoot running as a tool for rehabbing certain running injuries. For example, in his book *Smart Running*, well-known author and coach Hal Higdon recommends barefoot running on sand or grass as a tool for treating plantar fasciitis. Higdon writes, "My theory was that with no shoes to cushion the blows, my body would be more sensitive to what the foot was doing as it touched the ground. Barefoot running worked for me, and I still believe that runners should include some barefoot running in their training to help strengthen their feet." Few, however, have recommended barefoot running as a full-time practice.

In some parts of the world, though, barefoot running remains the default. For example, many elite East African runners spend their childhood running barefoot, and debate abounds as to whether this is a contributing factor to their distance running prowess. For example, former marathon world record holder Haile Gebrselassie of Ethiopia told CNN in an interview: "When I had no shoes I was comfortable—I used to run barefoot. When I wore shoes it was difficult. To run in shoes was OK, but at the beginning of my career it was hard. In our countryside, you see those kids they are very comfortable with no shoes. It's better to have no shoes than not the right ones."

The comfort, grace, and speed with which children in Africa run in their bare feet was emphasized in an essay by Adharanand Finn titled "Young, Barefoot and Fiercely Competitive: Kenya's Future Athletes" and published in *The Guardian* in early 2011. Finn spent six months living and training in the town of Iten, Kenya with the goal of figuring out just what makes Kenyan distance runners so dominant in international-level competition. The most commonly cited reason put forth by the Kenyan runners he met was their extremely active childhood. "Most run long distances to school each morning, and when they get home they are sent out to tend to the goats or sheep," Finn reports. "There are few televisions, let alone PlayStations or Xboxes." Quite simply, good habits developed in youth can pay big dividends later on in life.

While in Kenya, Finn had the opportunity to observe a children's cross-country race. He marveled at the number of elite runners who showed up to watch the kids run, and was impressed by the level of effort put forth by the youngsters. "Every single child runs as though possessed," writes Finn, "they charge like mini racehorses around the course. Even the children right at the back are pushing along at a decent pace." He goes on to observe that ". . . virtually all the children are running barefoot. Barefoot running is a growing trend in the West, based on the theory that conventional running shoes force you to run in an inefficient and injury-inducing style. It's interesting to note that here the only children wearing running shoes are at the very back of the field." Finn continues, saying that "In one race, the further back in the field the girls finish, the better their shoes, to the absurd extent that the girl with the newest, sleekest running shoes of all comes in last, while the girl whose shoes are only slightly worse finishes second to last." And what, you might ask, is the reward for the barefoot winners of each race? "Ironically," reports Finn, "the prize . . . is a pair of Nike running trainers."

If even a small part of the distance-running prowess of the Kenyan elites could be attributed to running barefoot when they were kids, it's tempting to ask whether the practice of putting children in miniature versions of adult running shoes from a very early age might have some kind of detrimental effect on their running potential. Do children really need heavy, cushioned shoes with built-in stability features? In a 2010 article titled "Growing Up Shod" in *Running Times Magazine*, Editor-in-Chief Jonathan Beverly quotes the head of the American Academy of Podiatric Sports Medicine as stating that "Kids should not be running in 'minimalist footwear' at all and, as in other shoes, should be wearing brand name running shoes with good motion control, cushioning, etc." Beverly is skeptical, writing that ". . . putting kids in motion-control shoes before they demonstrate the need for them feels like prescribing corrective eyeglasses to all children as soon as they start to read." Furthermore, Beverly continues, "The thousands of East African youth running miles to school barefoot argue . . . against the idea that shoes are necessary to prevent injury, and the resulting stride they develop speaks for itself in terms of running results."

Does this mean that all parents should have their children toss away their shoes or donate them to Goodwill and spend their days barefoot? Beverly isn't willing to go that far, pointing out that barefoot running can be a challenge due to lack of suitable running surfaces, and because a child that has grown up shod is likely to have adapted to shoes to a certain degree (more on this to come). He does, however, suggest that parents "encourage kids to go barefoot whenever possible." When barefoot is not an option, Beverly recommends that parents "Buy the most minimal shoes appropriate for your child. Look for low heel height, low-profile cushioning, flexibility (in the right place, at the ball of the foot), light weight, ample toe room. Often the minimal choice will be general-use shoes rather than running specific shoes, which tend to be designed as mini-adult, cushioned stability trainers." Beverly goes on to quote podiatrist Paul Langer, chair of the American Academy of Podiatric Sports Medicine's Footwear Committee, who cautiously says that "While research does not yet allow us to predict the long-term risks/benefits of minimalist footwear in children, it does suggest that allowing the feet and lower extremities to develop naturally with minimal cushioning or support is ideal."

How exactly might growing up in shoes impact one's ability to become a fleet-footed and efficient runner? Let's start with biomechanics. Since barefoot is the default human condition (we come out of the womb without shoes!), then any deviation from the natural state could have consequences. Beverly again quotes podiatrist Paul Langer, who emphasizes that scientific studies have shown that ". . . our feet are sensory organs that allow us to interact with our environment and to develop natural movement patterns. These studies suggest that shoes can interfere with that development. Balance, stride length and stride width are all influenced by our ability to sense the surface we are landing on. Clearly, the more "stuff" between the foot and the ground the less ability we have to sense the landing surface."

Wearing shoes removes your feet from direct contact with the surface below. So the messages coming in from the sensory structures in your soles get garbled, and you begin to move in a different way. Put simply, shoes can alter how you walk and run. Physical therapist and University of Virginia gait lab director Jay Dicharry likes to think of footwear as a filter that can interfere with normal sensory perception. "If you add a filter, you change the response of the body. The shoe affects the internal muscle response. If there's a poor stabilization response by the body (because of a particular shoe), then that overloads the body's tissue and then you get breakdown."

It might seem like a simple and straightforward task to determine how footwear might modify your running form. Run with shoes on, then run without them—and compare! The problem with this approach is that movement patterns, once ingrained, can be difficult to alter. If you spend most of your life walking and running in shoes, it might not be easy to suddenly adapt on the spot to an entirely new condition. In his book *Run Fast: How to Beat Your Best Time Every Time*, Hal Higdon discusses how exercise physiologist Dr. David Costill believes that motor patterns developed early in life can become "frozen," and that while minor adjustments might be possible, major changes are unlikely. As an analogy, Costill cites his experience with swimming, saying "You learn a smooth stroke early, or you never learn." In other words, if you don't learn how to run properly at a young age, it might be very difficult to learn how to run properly later on in life. Despite Costill's doubts, recent research on gait retraining via real-time feedback does seem to suggest that form change in running is indeed possible, at least to some degree, but that it might not happen all at once. A better way to examine the effects of shoes is to look at runners who have *never* worn them—like the youths who Adharanand Finn described as being at the front-of-the-pack in races he observed during his time in Kenya.

Dr. Daniel Lieberman, one of the pioneers of the Persistence Hunting/Running Man Theory that we covered in the first chapter, has a strong personal and academic interest in ancestral human (and thus, barefoot) running. In fact, the media often calls the Harvard anthropologist "the barefoot professor," because he too likes to run barefoot. Lieberman wanted to get a better idea of what running form untainted by footwear might look like, so he traveled to Kenya's Rift Valley, a place inhabited by a sizable population of people who have never worn shoes. Lieberman filmed both adolescent and adult runners, some of whom were regular shoe wearers, and others who were habitually barefoot. What Lieberman observed during his time in Africa was striking: almost every habitually unshod runner (those who had never worn shoes) ran in a way that is rarely seen in the shod world. Instead of contacting the ground on the rearfoot, or what we more commonly call the heel, the vast majority of Lieberman's habitually unshod Kenyan runners contacted the ground on the midfoot, along the entire outer margin of the foot, or the forefoot, on the pad just behind the base of the little toe. Based on this research, Lieberman and his colleagues published their findings in a 2010 issue of the journal *Nature*. Their study also revealed that:

1. Kenyans who had grown up barefoot but started wearing shoes later in life most often landed on the forefoot when running barefoot, but showed mixed footstrike patterns when wearing shoes (forefoot landing was still most common).
2. Adolescent Kenyans who had grown up wearing shoes tended to rearfoot strike in both the shod and unshod conditions, though their rearfoot strike was less pronounced (i.e., flatter footplant) when barefoot.
3. American runners who regularly run barefoot or in minimal footwear lacking arch support and cushioning also landed most frequently on their forefoot when running barefoot, but some reverted back to a rearfoot striking form when wearing shoes.
4. Americans who regularly wear shoes when running almost always land on their heel, regardless of whether they were shod or barefoot. Like the habitually shod Kenyans, the rearfoot strike was less pronounced when barefoot.

When asked to comment about these results, Lieberman emphasized that in all categories there is some amount of variability. "Barefoot runners sometimes rearfoot strike, and shod runners sometimes forefoot strike, and why runners land sometimes one way or another probably is affected by many factors such as speed, fatigue, surface, and so on."

Lieberman wasn't the first scientist to study barefoot running, and there is a lot more that differentiates barefoot from shod running form than simply the location where the foot makes initial contact with the ground (more on this in later chapters). However, what was unique about his work was that he was the first to document foot strike patterns in barefoot runners who had never before worn shoes, and in doing so he provided a tantalizing glimpse at how humans might have run in the absence of footwear.

Following in the (barefoot) footsteps of Christopher McDougall's wildly popular book *Born to Run*, Lieberman's publication came out at a time when the topic of barefoot running was red hot. As a result of such coincidental timing, the influence of Lieberman's work was immense. The media latched on, putting out story after story proclaiming the benefits of running barefoot. Based upon the level of coverage, one would have thought that runners everywhere had tossed their shoes and were now padding down streets and trails in their bare feet. The reality, however, is that the uniqueness of the story drove the media coverage far more than actual level of participation on the part of runners. Much to Lieberman's dismay, many of the media reports that came out carried with them either implicit or explicit suggestions that his research showed that running barefoot reduces injury risk—it did not, and Lieberman himself has made this point repeatedly. As a result of repeated misrepresentation of his findings, Lieberman posted the following statement on the Harvard University website dedicated to his barefoot running work: "Please note that we present no data on how people should run, whether shoes cause some injuries, or whether barefoot running causes other kinds of injuries. We believe there is a strong need for controlled, prospective studies on these issues."

Lieberman simply showed that you run differently when you take your shoes off, and suggested that the reason was related to the fact that it hurts to heel strike when running on a hard, tough surface. He did not, however, look at injury risk, and as the above statement attests, he views the relative benefits of shod compared to unshod running from an injury standpoint to be an open question deserving of further investigation.

Because media hype often carries more weight than scientific reality with the public at large, an increasing number of runners started to experiment with barefoot and minimalist running. And many did so without considering the risks inherent in making a dramatic change in how they ran—this despite repeated warnings coming from those with plenty of experience running without shoes.

As we have previously noted, rapid changes in training methods or footwear styles can stress the body in ways that it's not used to, and in the process increase the risk of injury until adaptations to the new stress are made. Running barefoot or in barefoot-style shoes is a dramatic change from what most people are used to, and a slow progression to the new style is well-advised.

Even Lieberman himself provided detailed tips on how to transition to barefoot or barefoot-style running on the Harvard website mentioned earlier. In particular, he emphasized the need to transition gradually:

> *Forefoot striking barefoot or in minimal footwear requires you to use muscles in your feet (mostly in the arch) that are probably very weak. Running this way also requires much more strength in your calf muscles than heel striking because these muscles must contract eccentrically (while lengthening) to ease the heel onto the ground following the landing. Novice forefoot and midfoot strikers typically experience tired feet, and very stiff, sore calf muscles. In addition, the Achilles tendon often gets very stiff. This is normal and eventually goes away, but you can do several things to make the transition successfully.*

"Build up slowly!" cautions Lieberman—rush matters, and you risk injury. "If you vigorously work out any weak muscles in your body, they will be sore and stiff. Your foot and calf muscles will be no exception. So please, don't overdo it because you will probably injure yourself if you do too much too soon."

Despite these cautionary words, more than a few runners failed to heed advice to proceed slowly. Always quick to try out the next great thing in order to improve their training or minimize injury risk, some runners shed their shoes or changed to ultraminimal footwear without significantly scaling back mileage. Others opted to try and immediately force an exaggerated forefoot strike rather than let the body adapt gradually because they had heard that was how one is supposed to run when barefoot. The result was predictable—people began showing up on Internet forums complaining of foot injuries like metatarsal stress fractures and the dreaded "top of foot pain," and podiatrists and physical therapists started reporting marked increases in the number of injured barefoot and minimalist runners visiting their clinics. These runners had jumped on the "free the feet" bandwagon without much thought or planning, and many unfortunately paid the price.

In particular, metatarsal stress fractures in the foot seem to be one of the most commonly reported injuries among new barefoot and minimalist runners, and Lieberman has some thoughts on why this might be the case:

{Stress fractures in the foot} generally occur on the second metatarsal, which is the most common foot fracture in shod runners as well. There are no solid studies on relative incidence rates yet, but it's clear that metatarsal fractures occur in both barefoot-minimalist runners and shod runners. According to the scientific literature, 90 percent of foot fractures are the second metatarsal, and that's all data from shod runners. One possibility is that we're seeing more metatarsal fractures in barefoot runners because there are more barefoot runners. I don't know yet if it's more prevalent.

{Metatarsal stress fractures} are probably not from landing because no barefoot runner lands on the second metatarsal. You land on the fourth and fifth metatarsal, and because the impact forces are so low, that's probably why those metatarsals are not getting fractured. But I do think that the problem, and this is just a hypothesis here, is that the second metatarsal fractures we are seeing are caused during toe-off, because it's during toe-off when you place peak forces on that part of the foot. Stress is force per unit area—if you're pushing off hard on a shoe, you're going to push off with the whole base of the shoe, so that's going to have a low stress. But if you're barefoot and pushing off hard, the area over which you're going to be pushing is vastly reduced so the stresses are going to go way up. Stresses go up and things break. That's because stress causes strain, and strain causes things to break. People who don't have the strength, they're pushing too hard, probably running too fast, and that might explain what some of the problems are.

The way to cure that, if you're really worried about it, is to wear a shoe. There are lots of minimal shoes you can wear that give you the same benefits of any other shoe. People have probably been forefoot striking for millennia in shoes and they were probably not breaking their metatarsals any more than anybody else. So if that's an issue for you, wear a shoe.

Lieberman goes on to express frustration about the exuberance with which some runners have taken to barefoot and minimalist running, and tempers the belief held by some barefooters that the practice is a cure-all for running injuries:

One of my big worries all along has been that people are going to injure themselves because they get excited and caught up in the hype. If you've ever looked at our {Harvard lab} website, every page screams 'do this carefully' and 'slowly and gradually' and 'if it hurts don't do it.' But people get very excited, you know, they read Chris McDougall's book and they think that if they run barefoot, everything in their life will become better, their teeth will become whiter, they'll get more girlfriends. Of course, runners are going to get injured, and barefoot runners are going to be no different than shod runners. I think they're probably just trading off one set of injuries for another.

Interestingly, Lieberman questions whether the recent rise of barefoot running-related injuries is caused by anything more than an increase in the number of barefoot runners. "The fact of the matter right now is that there's no data. You can quote a podiatrist who says that there's a rash of injuries, which of course there is because there's now a rash of barefoot runners," says Lieberman. "What we don't yet know is what the costs versus the benefits are. We desperately need careful, prospective studies."

The question of whether or not runners should consider running barefoot is a contentious one to say the least, and debates among bloggers, health professionals, coaches, and academics about the merits of barefoot running can at times get downright hostile. Unfortunately, some people will never change their opinions on the subject, particularly the most ardent of the pro- and anti- barefoot running camps. Given this "standoff," it's worth discussing some challenges faced by the barefoot runner.

Challenge #1: Shoes Alter Our Feet and Legs

One of the biggest potential challenges faced by a habitually shod runner who decides to give barefooting a shot is the very real likelihood that their feet have been altered from natural human shape and function by chronic use of ill-fitting footwear. In other words, feet of modern runners in the developed world are probably quite a bit different from those of the Kenyan adolescents that Lieberman filmed who had never previously worn shoes in their lives.

It's fairly well established that living a shod life can alter the anatomy and function of our feet. For example, a paper published in 2009 in the journal *Footwear Science* reports fascinating results from a study conducted by a group headed by Kristiaan D'Aout from the University of Antwerp in Belgium. The researchers traveled to southern India and made anatomical measurements of the feet of habitually shod and habitually unshod individuals. They also took measurements from a group of Belgians for comparative purposes, since even the typically shod Indians wear mostly non-constrictive shoes like sandals (they also typically go barefoot as children). In addition to the foot examination, the researchers had each individual walk over a pressure mat to examine how pressure is applied to the sole of the foot during normal walking.

What the researchers found was that the habitually barefoot group had the widest feet, and both groups of Indians had longer feet when corrected for overall body size than the Belgians. In other words, the Belgians had short, scrawny feet compared to the Indians. When they looked at pressure distributions under the feet during walking, they found that the habitually barefoot group used more of the foot surface to disperse pressure (particularly in the region of the midfoot), whereas the Belgians tended to exhibit stronger and more localized pressure peaks under the heel and under the second and third metatarsal heads (recall that the second metatarsal is the most commonly fractured metatarsal in runners, both shod and probably barefoot). The authors concluded in their report: "The evolutionary history of humans shows that barefoot walking is the biologically natural situation. The use of footwear remains necessary, especially on unnatural substrates, in athletics, and in some pathologies, but current data suggests that footwear that fails to respect natural foot shape and function will ultimately alter the morphology and the biomechanical behavior of the foot."

Other studies have examined skeletal remains from medieval Europe in comparison to later time periods and have found that foot conditions like hallux valgus (when the big toe is bent inward toward the other toes, and often associated with a bunion) appear in concert with rising popularity of shoes with narrow, pointed toeboxes and/or stiff leather boots. For example, in a 2007 paper in the journal *Joint Bone Spine*, Bertrand Mafart of the National Museum of Natural History in France concludes that:

The increase in the prevalence of hallux valgus over time suggests an influence of changes in footwear. The heeled shoes and boots made of stiff leather that men wore in premodern times probably promoted the development of hallux valgus. However, the prevalence of hallux valgus in women in western industrialized countries today is even higher than that in our historical population of older premodern individuals, suggesting an extremely deleterious effect of contemporary female footwear.

One need look no further than the feet of a modern woman with a *Sex and the City* penchant for fashionable high-heeled shoes to see the effects that a constricting, pointed toebox can have on the shape of the foot.

Despite the frequency with which even modern humans choose narrow shoes with pointed toes, the negative impacts of such a design have been recognized among shoemakers for centuries. For example, in his 1885 treatise titled "*The Art of Boot and Shoemaking, A Practical Handbook,*" John Bedford Leno writes the following:

> {. . . *pointed toe boots are an abomination, false in theory, false practically, and destructive, not only of the ease and comfort of those that wear them, but, sooner or later, of their walking powers.*
>
> *In the natural foot when off duty, its toes touch each other gently; when called on to assist locomotion or bear their share of the superincumbent weight, they spread out though not to any great extent, it is true. This being their natural action, no sensible maker of boots and shoes would attempt to restrain it, or allow it to be restrained. Still, from a want of knowledge of the foot's anatomical structure, the stupid mandates of all-powerful fashion, the folly of maker and wearer, or from one cause or many, it has been restrained, and as a necessary consequence, few feet widen to the extent that is required. What chance is there of the toes of a vast number of feet spreading when instead of remaining side by side as nature intended they should lie, they have been so crushed and crowded together that they literally overlie each other? Again, it may be said that the grand lesson taught by Anatomy is the danger of allowing undue pressure to interfere with the foot's action, or rather multiplicity of actions.*

Which "actions" might be hampered by feet that have been deformed by constricting toe boxes? For one, proper positioning and stabilizing function of the big toe when the foot is in contact with the ground is critical to your ability to maintain balance, both while standing and while on the move. In fact, proper stabilizing function of the big toe is one of the traits that Jay Dicharry points to as critical for all runners. He feels that improved ability to balance on one leg during the stance phase of running could help runners reduce their risk of succumbing to a host of repetitive stress injuries.

While fashion is often to blame for society's willingness to indulge itself with extravagant, ill-fitting footwear, John Bedford Leno also believed that shoemakers of his day shared some portion of the blame. In particular, he chastises them for failing to understand the anatomy and function of the human foot:

> *Shoemakers as a rule, it must be confessed, know little of the foot's anatomy. At a time like the present, when the value of technical education is so generally recognized, it singular that no satisfactory effort is being made to relieve them of this disadvantage, Naturally it may be thought that this would have been the first thing taught in the art and mystery of boot and shoemaking, for how is it possible that a maker of these necessary articles, void of such knowledge, can properly furnish the foot?*

The scenario is not all that different today, especially within the athletic footwear industry. Job qualifications in athletic shoe design tend more toward those who have experience with fashion and industrial design than those with a detailed understanding of the anatomy and biomechanics of the human foot. Though some companies carry out extensive biomechanical testing and research on shoes that are in development, industry insiders often lament off the record that the best shoe for the foot may not always be the best shoe for the market, and the market is ultimately where profit is made.

One place where footwear function takes firm precedence over fashion is in the military, where an ill-fitting boot could be all it takes to remove an otherwise able-bodied soldier from the battlefield. Napoleon might have said that an army marches on its stomach, but it still needs to be wearing the right kind of footwear. Indeed, recognition of the deforming effects of footwear and their consequences to proper foot function has long been a topic of interest in the armed forces. In 1912, Edward Lyman Munson, then president of the United States Army Shoe Board, set out to design a new boot for the nation's soldiers that would better serve their foot health. In the end, he came with the boot shape, or "last," that served U.S. army soldiers through the Second World War.

In his 1912 book "*The Soldier's Foot and the Military Shoe*," Munson points out that "the amount of disability from foot injury in modern armies is enormous," but contends that ". . . because foot injuries have usually been so common among soldiers of all armies is no reason for our accepting them with patient resignation as one of the inevitable concomitants of field service." Munson viewed ill-fitting boots to be a major contributing factor to the high number of foot injuries seen in soldiers, and he emphasized that their shoes rarely match the actual anatomical shape of their feet:

The human foot is not to be regarded, as seems almost to be the idea with many, as an incoordinating mass of flesh, bone and gristle which may with impunity be crowded into almost any sort of protective covering to form a fleshy peg, more or less similar to a horse's hoof, on which to walk. It is, on the contrary, one of the most intricate anatomical structures of the human body.

Munson was by no means against shoes. Rather, he felt that ill-fitting shoes combined with the more sedentary nature of individuals in modern civilization did serious harm to their feet. He writes, "The introduction of railroads, street cars and automobiles, has materially interfered with foot development in many. And with the lesser need for the use of the foot in walking, came the introduction of deforming and confining shoe types, by which the use of certain foot muscles was interfered with and their consequent atrophy and weakening was inevitable." He saves some of his harshest criticism for makers of fashionable shoes for civilian use:

The construction of shoes for civilians is influenced almost wholly by considerations of fashion and style. These are irrational and are frequently changed in the financial interest of the shoe trade. The lasts are devised by persons grossly ignorant of, and quite indifferent to, the structure of the human foot and its physiological requirements as to covering. Shoes built upon them range through every degree of the bizarre and represent the most amazing conceptions of their originators as to the diverse shapes which the human foot should be forced to assume.

It is rare to find in civil life a shoe that even approaches the normal foot in shape and contour. Few manufacturers make them, as they are not salable to the general public, whose choice is swayed rather by considerations of fashion than comfort . . . The shoe trade considers itself free from blame, as it is frankly in the business for profit, and is interested in giving the public what the latter thinks it wants.

{. . . all but a very few civilians are so influenced by the subtle suggestive influences of manufacturers' styles as largely to disregard matters of fit, shape and comfort, and tend to buy the enormities which the shoe manufacturers

think it to be in their interest to put on the market. The very few who, despite such influences, would tend to prefer sensible shoes, receive little encouragement and frequently are quite unable to find stock in what they would like to purchase. A vicious circle is thus created, under which civilian shoe manufacturers and shoe wearers seem to vie with each other in injuring the feet. Add to this the firm resolve of nearly every civilian to crowd the foot into the narrowest and shortest shoe that it can be forced into without severe suffering, and the evil results to the foot are tremendously increased. The result is that practically every soldier in the army has had his feet more or less injured by the shoes he wore before entering the services; and that bad feet, especially in city bred applicants, have come to be one of the chief causes for rejection for enlistment.

When considering the writings of both Munson and Leno, what's fascinating is that very little has changed in terms of the typical shape mismatch between shoe and foot. Just like it was in the late 1800s and early 1900s, narrow-width casual shoes with a pointed toebox are still quite the norm for both men and women. This approach to footwear construction applies equally to running shoes, where until very recently an actual foot-shaped shoe such as those made by industry newcomer Altra Running out of Utah was nearly impossible to find.

It is probable that just as few soldiers of Munson's day entered the army without preexisting foot problems, few individuals in modern society can enter into barefoot or barefoot-style running without some form of foot weakness (bony or muscular) or deformity caused by chronic shoe wear. Certainly, even fewer will have feet resembling anything close to those found in habitually unshod populations like those in India or Kenya. Furthermore, the fact that shoe-induced deformities have been known for centuries makes it highly likely that even runners who used the stripped down shoes that were the norm prior to the advent of the modern running shoe in the latter half of the twentieth century were doing so with feet that were quite divergent from those who grew up barefoot—as Munson pointed out, fashionable shoes for all-day use have long diverged in shape from any semblance of the actual anatomy of human foot. Rather than create shoes to match our anatomy, we alter our anatomy to fit our shoes. We've got it all backwards! The result is that most of us run on feet that are far removed in anatomy and function from those of our persistence-hunting ancestors, and it should therefore come as little surprise when some individuals encounter trouble when trying to transition to running without shoes or in minimalist footwear—their feet are simply not adapted to running in their default state.

Chronic use of anatomically inappropriate footwear can have effects that extend beyond just the feet. For example, Robert Csapo of the University of Vienna and a team of researchers at Manchester Metropolitan University in the U.K. decided to examine the effects of habitual wearing of high-heeled shoes on women's calf muscles and Achilles tendons. In a 2010 paper published in the *Journal of Experimental Biology*, they reported the results of a study in which they compared aspects of lower leg anatomy between a group of eleven women who wore stilettos (minimum heel height of 5 centimeters) for an average of sixty hours per week for two years, to a group of nine women who wore "flat" shoes most of the time (averaging only about two hours of stiletto wear per week). Using a variety of medical imaging (such as MRI and ultrasonography), as well as strength-testing techniques, they determined that the high heel aficionados had shorter fascicles (bundles of muscle fibers) in the gastrocnemius muscle in their calves, and thicker, stiffer Achilles tendons. The shorter calf muscle fibers and loss of springiness in the Achilles tendon combined to reduce the range of motion at the ankle joint. The authors suggested that this combination of outcomes could explain why many women who habitually wear high-heeled shoes complain of muscular soreness when switching to flats.

Interestingly, one of the most common complaints from runners after an initial attempt to run barefoot or in flat, barefoot-style shoes is extreme soreness in the calf muscles. It's not a huge leap to consider that wearing shoes with even a modest heel lift (as found even on most men's work, casual, and athletic shoes) might impact the anatomy of the calf muscle and Achilles tendon in ways that can make running barefoot difficult, at least for a time. It's often overlooked, but it's probably more likely that what you wear on your feet for most of the day is going to have a greater long-term impact on foot and leg function than what you wear when you run. Consider this the next time you slide on your favorite pumps, oxfords, or even steel-toed boots before heading off to work—although variable in height, all typically have a fairly sizable heel lift.

Barefoot Running and Joint Torques

The effects of footwear are not solely limited to anatomical changes like bent toes and shortened tendons—they can also alter the biomechanics of how one runs. Dr. Casey Kerrigan is one of the world's leading experts on the effects of footwear on gait. She has published over ninety scientific papers on human walking and running gaits, and she founded the gait labs at both Harvard University and the University of Virginia. The goal of much of her research has been to attempt to elucidate the causes of overuse injuries and long-term degenerative joint disorders like osteoarthritis. She has come to believe that poorly designed shoes are potentially a significant contributor to lower extremity joint woes.

In a study published in 2009 in the journal *Physical Medicine and Rehabilitation (PM&R)*, Kerrigan and colleagues sought to document how joint torques changed when subjects ran in typical running shoes versus when they ran barefoot. The researchers (including physical therapist Jay Dicharry) studied sixty-eight runners on a high-tech treadmill capable of measuring forces underfoot, and simultaneously filmed them with a 10 camera, three-dimensional motion analysis system. Each individual ran both barefoot and in a pair of Brooks Adrenaline running shoes, which are classified as a stability shoe with a raised heel that is about 12 mm higher than the forefoot, arch support, and a dual-density midsole (softer foam on the lateral side, firmer on the medial side) intended to limit overpronation.

For those without a background in physics, engineering, or biomechanics, a torque is simply a force that rotates an object around some type of axis. Torques are dependent on two factors: the magnitude of the force applied, and the distance at which the force is applied relative to the point of rotation. For a familiar example, when you use a wrench to twist a stuck nut, your likelihood of loosening the nut is dependent on how hard you push or pull on the wrench handle, and how long the handle of the wrench is. More strength applied to a longer handled wrench is more likely to free up the nut. In a similar manner, when your foot is in contact with the ground, the ground reaction force (GRF), which is the force exerted by the ground back onto the foot, extends away from the ground toward the body. The calculations are complex, but the magnitude and direction of the GRF can be determined through use of a force plates embedded into the ground or underneath a treadmill belt. The larger the GRF and the greater the distance that it travels relative each joint center, the greater the torque that GRF applies to each joint. Assuming that joints are not going to simply collapse, muscular effort is required to resist joint torque caused by the GRF to keep one's joints stable.

The results of Kerrigan's study indicated that six of the nine joint torques that they calculated were significantly higher in the running shoe condition when compared to barefoot (the rest were not different between the conditions). Three joint torques increased considerably when runners wore the Brooks shoes. First, knee flexion torque increased by 36 percent; the authors observed that this "potentially increases the work of the quadriceps muscle, increases strain through the patella tendon, and increases pressure across the patellofemoral joint." Second, knee varus torque increased by 38 percent. Knee varus torque causes the knee to bend outward (bowlegging), and can lead to greater compression through the inner side of the knee joint, which is the most common site of degenerative damage in knee osteoarthritis. Third, hip internal rotation torque increased by 54 percent. Kerrigan suggested that the increased hip torque could represent a risk factor for hip osteoarthritis, and other studies have suggested that increases in this torque might contribute to knee injuries and iliotibial band syndrome. None of these changes are in and of themselves guaranteed to cause injury, but they do indicate that the forces applied around the knee and hip were higher when the runners were shod.

What caused the increase in joint torques observed by Kerrigan and her colleagues? Could it be a change in form when shoes are removed? Possibly, but the results showed that although stride length decreased when barefoot, stride length change wasn't strongly correlated with changes in torque between the conditions. Instead, they focused on the properties of the running shoes themselves—the elevated heel, arch support, and dual density midsole. For example, from previous research in their lab, they knew that adding additional arch material or a medial wedge can increase knee varus torque during both walking and running because they tend to shift pressure more toward the medial (arch) side of the foot. This medial pressure shift, in turn, alters the direction of the ground reaction force so that it passes further away from the knee joint, thus increasing the torque that causes bowlegging of the knee (remember, torque is dependent on both the magnitude of the force applied and its distance from the joint that it rotates).

Kerrigan's paper concluded by saying that although some studies have shown benefit of orthotics with medial posting for treatment of knee pain, "the design of current running shoes, with various heel-cushioning strategies and technologies to increase medial support to control foot pronation, has become widely accepted as the industry standard. However, there is no clinical evidence to support that this design is optimal to promote the long-term health of runners." They go on to encourage the ". . . development of new footwear designs that encourage or mimic the natural compliance that normal foot function provides while minimizing knee and hip joint torques . . . Reducing joint torques with footwear to that of barefoot running, while providing meaningful footwear functions, especially compliance, should be the goal of new footwear designs" (the term compliance refers here to compression and release of the shoe midsole).

Fed up with a market filled with what she feels are poorly designed shoes with foam midsoles that don't provide the necessary compliance that the body needs, Kerrigan resigned her tenured position as chair of the Department of Physical Medicine and Rehabilitation at the University of Virginia to start a shoe company called OESH with her husband, Robert Kusyk. Together, they had decided that she could have a more positive impact on foot and leg health by developing a new type of footwear rather than by spending her days in the clinic or publishing academic papers. Her first shoes were released in 2011, and possess a midsole composed of carbon fiber cantilevers instead of foam, with the specific goal of providing a sole that can compress and release in tune with the rise and fall of the mass of the body. Time will tell whether Kerrigan's decades of research have led to the creation of a shoe that will put a dent in the epidemic of joint injuries that plague so many people today.

In summary, it's important to note that the consequences of shoe-induced alterations in gait biomechanics or foot and leg anatomy to injury risk in runners are still not well understood, nor is there strong scientific evidence regarding precisely how much of any damage already incurred can be reversed via a change in footwear (or lack thereof). For example, can a woman regain natural form and function by ditching her stilettos in favor of more sensible shoes that respect foot anatomy? Possibly—anecdotes from individuals reporting alterations in foot shape as a result of adopting a more habitually barefoot lifestyle exist, and barefoot/minimalist runners typically see a lessening of calf soreness with time, but carefully documented case studies are hard to come by. Regardless, the potentially negative influence of anatomical acclimation to modern shoe styles suggests that any habitually shod individual who is considering making an abrupt switch to running barefoot or in very minimal footwear should do so with considerable caution.

Challenge #2: The Hard Surfaces Factor

In 1924, Arthur Newton sailed from South Africa to England in an attempt to set a world record in the 50-mile race. As an ultrarunner, Newton was accustomed to running 200 or more miles per week during peak training, but upon arriving in England he began to encounter some trouble with his legs. In his 1935 book *Running*, Newton described the worrisome situation:

> *In less than a fortnight I was pulled up again—it hadn't struck me that because the roads were hard (I had been used to unimproved country ones in Natal) I should have to get used to the new conditions. Anyhow, my shin and ankle swelled up and . . . after a week of only 116 miles the annoyance was well on its way to a finish."*
>
> *Thinking I was now pretty safe, I let out for a couple of weeks in the old style, 251 and 295 miles. The latter was certainly rather more than usual, but the roads were so good in comparison to what I had been used to that the extra mileage was not very noticeable. How the other leg must have chuckled to itself as it quietly prepared for a finisher . . . the left leg had already shown it wasn't going to stand any nonsense; the right wasn't going to be done out of its turn. Training dropped to some 60 per cent. (sic) of the normal, while I struggled along with a swollen and inflamed shin and ankle. No good, I couldn't shake it off, though I carried on like this for a month."*
>
> *I went to London to see a specialist. I was told that the trouble was due to the interminable vibration on muscles and sinews caused by the steady hammering of the feet on hard surfaced roads . . . I was advised to cut my daily run down to a dozen miles or so, and to attend every day for massage.*

The good news for Newton was that the unnamed specialist he consulted in London was able to help him manage his shin splints (if only we could all claim a daily 12 mile run to be therapy!), and he recovered well enough that he did indeed break the 50-mile record when race day arrived. But, what is perhaps most interesting about Newton's story is how the health specialist identified the actual source of his temporary affliction—the road surface. Newton had made a sudden change in his training by going from a softer to a harder surface. In fact, the topic of running surface is one that frequently comes up today in the context of the barefoot running debate, and is worthy of an in-depth discussion.

One of the most frequently posed objections to barefoot running in the modern world is that our ancestors didn't evolve to run on hard surfaces like asphalt and concrete. Rather, this argument goes, humans are built to run on softer, more natural surfaces like sand and grass, and thus barefoot running should be limited to this type of surface. The thinking is that soft, natural surfaces will reduce the impact that occurs when your feet hit the ground. Sounds reasonable, but what is the reality?

The notion that modern hard surfaces are atypical of ancestral running surfaces is challenged frequently by those who have run in areas in Africa where our species originated. For example, Daniel Lieberman reports that he's "done a lot of running in Africa, and most of Africa is not like a lawn or a beach. It's actually pretty hard." He feels that the surface hardness argument may be irrelevant since "the whole point about forefoot striking and midfoot striking, the way in which people run barefoot, is that it's low impact . . . barefoot runners will tell you that they couldn't care less about the hardness of the surface. What they care about is the roughness of the surface." Indeed, if you ask a barefoot runner about his or her favorite running surface, many will answer that it's smooth, clean asphalt, and not grass or sand. Although certainly harder and less forgiving than most natural surfaces (except maybe stone), smooth asphalt surfaces have the advantage of being very predictable, and it's very easy to see and avoid any debris that might be on the ground—the latter is more difficult when running on a grass surface or on a trail.

While the lack of variability in a hard asphalt surface raises the risk of repetitive stress injury, its predictability might just allow a runner to develop a more dialed-in stride for impact reduction purposes. Researchers have shown that when running, humans subconsciously tune their stride to the surface that they are running on. Benno Nigg, a biomechanist from the University of Calgary, believes that a runner tunes his or her muscular response to ground impact from step to step in order to minimize vibrations that pass through the soft tissues (muscles, tendons, ligaments) of the lower limbs.

Every time your foot makes contact with the ground when you run, the soft tissues in your legs jiggle or vibrate relative to the bones that they are attached to. Too much jiggling can damage these tissues and cause soreness, and thus the muscle tuning paradigm suggests that you automatically modify your muscular response to impact in order to minimize the jiggling. In this paradigm, impact acts as an input to tell the muscles what to do. For example, if impacts are hard, you tense up your muscles a bit to reduce the jiggle—thus, the tuning response will vary depending on the properties of the shoes and surfaces under your feet.

Applying this understanding to Arthur Newton's anecdote, one might hypothesize that when he went from running on poorly kept roads in South Africa to harder roads in England, one of the following things might have happened. First, the harder surface could have increased his soft tissue vibrations to a level that became damaging (as hypothesized by his doc, who appears to have been well ahead of his time in his thinking about the cause of running injuries!). Or, Newton unconsciously tuned his stride on the new surface to manage these vibrations, and simply did too much too soon with a movement or muscle activity pattern that he was not accustomed to.

Another thing that happens as you run is that you modify the stiffness of your lower limbs in order to maintain a relatively stable up-down displacement of your center of mass, which is located somewhere in the vicinity of your hips (you can think of stiffness as the amount of flex that occurs in the leg joints—less flex equals a stiffer joint). In this sense the mass of your body can be viewed as a weight, and your lower leg can be viewed as a spring that supports that weight—your body bounces up and down on your leg springs as you run, and this is known as the spring-mass model of running. Moving your body up and down while running is energetically costly—too much bouncing will tire you out faster, and, incidentally, this is also why carrying additional body weight makes you less efficient when you run. The body seems to have an inherent desire to control the vertical displacement of the center of mass (to control the bounce) in order to keep it as stable as possible regardless of what is happening underfoot. If viewing a runner from the side, this can be thought of as a relatively stable up-down position of the head and trunk regardless of the type of surface the runner might be passing over at any given moment.

To give you an extreme example of this, think about what would happen if you were to run across a hard gym floor and then onto a trampoline.
What would your legs do? Most probably, when you hit the trampoline
your joints would flex less than they did while running over the hard floor
(less range of motion), resulting in a stiffer leg. The springiness of the leg
is a largely a function of the movement of its major joints—the hip, knee,
ankle—as well as the actions of the muscles, tendons, and ligaments in
the legs and feet. As a general rule, leg stiffness will increase on softer
surfaces, and will decrease (the joints will bend more) on hard surfaces.
It is possible, however, that there may be a cost to extremes of stiffness
in either direction. Too straight a leg could increase impact through the
bones (think of the jolt you get when stepping unexpectedly off a curb),
whereas a leg with extreme bending at the joints could work the muscles
of the leg a lot harder (a wasteful, inefficient gait).

The mechanism by which these stiffness adaptations are accomplished
is not entirely understood, but it seems to happen on the fly, and most
of us are able to make the necessary changes prior to stepping on a new
type of surface if we know that a change in surface properties is coming.
Conversely, unexpected changes can cause trouble. In his 2010 book titled "*Biomechanics of Sport Shoes*," Benno Nigg tells an interesting story
about how he was able to help reduce injury rates among Cirque du Soleil
performers by applying his knowledge of how gait adapts to the surface
underfoot. He observed that the stage used by the performers consisted
of a pliable surface supported at regular intervals by hard beams. Viewed
from the top, the performers could not predict when they might step on
a softer, more pliable region or a hard region overlying one of the support beams. This made it very difficult for the performers to appropri-
ately pre-adapt their landings to the surface at any given location on the
stage. Somewhat surprisingly, his advice was to rebuild the stage with a
uniformly hard surface (a predictable surface). Yet a hard surface is not
what you might expect as the ideal stage surface for performers that do a
lot of running and jumping. After making the stage modifications suggested by Nigg, injury rates were reduced from 25 percent of performers
at any given time to 2 to 3 percent. This is a great example showing that
increasing surface hardness can actually reduce injury rates by increasing predictability, and provides insight into why many barefoot runners
claim that smooth asphalt is their favorite surface to run on. (If you'd

like to experience what it feels like to not be able to anticipate a change in surface hardness, find a safe spot where asphalt is located adjacent to grass. Close your eyes and run slowly from one surface onto the other. A bit unnerving isn't it!)

The amazing ability of the human body to adapt gait to surfaces of varying hardness has been further demonstrated by studies that have actually measured impact forces on these differing surfaces. Quite surprisingly, several studies have shown that impact force actually does not differ when running on soft vs. hard surfaces—one study published by podiatrist Raymond Feehery in 1986 found that peak impact forces were actually slightly higher on grass than on concrete, though the rate of force application was reduced. Furthermore, some injury studies have found no significant effect of running surface on likelihood of sustaining a running injury. For example, Stephen Walter and colleagues from McMaster University report in a 1989 issue of the *Archives of Internal Medicine* that "frequency of running on asphalt, concrete, grass, or dirt" had no significant relationship to injury risk. Furthermore, a study headed by Caroline Macera of the University of South Carolina in the same issue of the *Archives of Internal Medicine* reports an increased risk of injury in female runners on concrete sidewalks, but a similar pattern was not found for males. There's certainly more work that needs to be done on the surface hardness issue. For example, it would be interesting to know whether the lack of pliability (or forgiveness) in an asphalt or concrete surface increases stress on the metatarsals during pushoff and thus might contribute to increasing risk of stress fractures. However, to date there is no clear, conclusive evidence that hardness of running surfaces in the modern world is a primary contributor to injury, or that it should be a barrier to the practice of barefoot running.

Challenge #3: Attack of the Stray Hypodermic Needle

Another frequent claim made by barefoot-running skeptics is that the risk of stepping on something dangerous is too high to make unshod running worth the risk. This argument tends to be overplayed and overblown— how often have you run along sidewalks strewn with medical waste? But one should not discount the risk posed by ground debris. For one thing, crushed rocks and pebbles tend to be pointy, and they tend to inflict pain when you step on them—it's not a pleasant feeling, even when wearing an ultraminimal shoe that offers some degree of protection. Natural debris like acorns or other nuts can also be a nuisance. Furthermore, who hasn't seen a broken bottle scattered on the sidewalk from time to time? Sure, it's easy enough to step around debris like this, but many runners would rather keep their head up and enjoy their surroundings as they run rather than focus on the ground so as to avoid stepping on something that might cause harm. Shoes let you check out and let the mind roam free when you feel like it, and sometimes this is just as desirable as the opposite extreme of being totally in tune with what is happening underfoot.

Some barefoot proponents go so far as to suggest that elites could do just as well, or potentially even better, if they simply ditched their shoes, since less weight on the feet correlates with higher running efficiency. For elites to do this makes no sense, and it goes beyond the fact that these runners are sponsored by shoe companies. If your paycheck depends on performing well and avoiding injury, why take the risk of stepping on something that might hurt you, or potentially end your career, even if that risk is limited? In his book *The Perfect Mile*, author Neal Bascomb recounts the story of legendary Australian miler John Landy, who stepped on a discarded flashbulb while training barefoot on grass just prior to his head-to-head showdown with Roger Bannister at the British Empire Games in 1954. Landy suffered a deep wound—severe enough to require stitches, but that didn't stop him from competing despite the pain. Though Landy ultimately still broke 4:00 in the race, Bannister wound up winning the much anticipated matchup, and we'll never know for sure how much of a role the barefoot running mishap might have played in the result. Such occurrences might be rare, but for an elite runner the risk is real enough to make barefoot running a risky prospect except under the safest of conditions.

Conclusion

There are a variety of other challenges that face the aspiring barefoot runner—social stigma, infections/parasites, heat/cold, and so forth—but despite these potential difficulties, some individuals have had great success running barefoot full-time. For example, Barefoot Ken Bob Saxton has run over seventy marathons without shoes. Some barefoot runners do it out of simple preference and a desire to better connect with the ground, whereas others do it because it has proven to be the only way that they can run without getting injured. However, most habitually barefoot runners will admit that there are occasions where shoes are necessary, even if they are nothing more than foot-gloves or strips of leather lashed to their soles.

Barefoot running has many merits and quite vocal advocates, but although it is becoming more accepted as a valid option for runners, the practice of full-time barefoot running will never be common. Runners love their shoes, and in many instances shoes are a necessity. Given this, we feel it might be instructive to now take a jog through the history of footwear, from the most basic forms from deep in the past, all the way to the modern running shoe of today.

⌘

CHAPTER 4

༄༅༈

The Running Shoe

I would advise that each runner leave shoes and stockings at home, but of course this should be optional with the individual; next to bare feet are sandals, next to sandals moccasins, next to moccasins, soft, low shoes.

—J. WILLIAM LLOYD, WHO IN 1890 WROTE
THE FIRST TREATISE ON RUNNING

Man spent several million years evolving as a runner. The athletic shoe has a much shorter history—about 180 years. But the modern running shoe is even younger, a mere adolescent who came of age during the early era of space exploration. The timing probably explains why Nike's original waffle-tread shoes that market-launched in 1972 became widely known as "moon shoes." The distinctive grid-like pattern that the soles made in dirt resembled the footprints left behind by the American astronauts on the lifeless, chalky lunar soil. Those NASA tread marks are still visible on the moon—untouched and undisturbed on the windless landscape. Yet here on our own planet, the evidence of where and how man first went shod is more difficult to nail down with any certainty. It's a guessing game with science helping when it can.

In 1938, Luther Cressman, an Oregon-based anthropologist who was once briefly married to Margaret Mead, unearthed a pair of well-preserved, shredded sagebrush bark sandals from an upraised volcanic landmass, also called a tuff ring, near Fort Rock, Oregon. These shoes were radiocarbon-dated to be around 10,000 years old, making them the oldest footwear ever discovered. Cressman ended up finding dozens of sandals buried beneath a hardened layer of volcanic ash that resulted from the eruption of the Mt. Mazama volcano 7,500 years ago. It was an amazing footwear fossil trove, but there is another coincidental item regarding this discovery that occasionally surfaces in books and articles about Nike's storied past. The University of Oregon's legendary track coach and co-founder of Nike, Bill Bowerman, who had created the original waffle trainer, was born in Fossil, Oregon, which is located about 150 miles north of the archeological site.

Bowerman's son, Jon, now in his early seventies and a former U.S. Olympic ski coach, still lives in Fossil on the family ranch that once bordered the infamous, scandal-plagued Bhagwan Rajneesh commune. In 2010, an important relic was found in a rubbish-filled landfill on the Bowerman ranch. Jon's brother accidentally came across the very same waffle iron that was used by his father to create a new urethane running sole. The iron was corroded, rusted, and clearly unusable.

Reached at his home in Fossil in December 2010, Jon Bowerman recalled that simple cooking gadget. "The chrome waffle iron had been in our family for a long time, since about 1936. It was either a wedding gift, or bought around the same time. It was small, so you could only make one waffle at a time. Which meant, Dad had to cook the rubber twice to make two soles. He then glued both soles to nylon uppers to make the final shoes."

Understandably, a whole lot of mythology has burnished this simple cooking appliance that should have its own display case in the Smithsonian, even though its closer-to-home final resting place is Nike's corporate headquarters in Beaverton, Oregon. The waffle iron actually belonged to Bill's wife. Years before oxidizing rust set in, the cooked, blackened rubber forever ruined the gadget. But what else do we know about the Bowerman waffle-iron legacy?

Two smartly written books, *Swoosh*, by J. B. Strasser and Laurie Becklund, and *Bill Bowerman and the Men of Oregon*, by Kenny Moore, make for fascinating reading about Bowerman and Nike's early history. Bowerman was a born tinkerer, blessed with the DNA of a restless, curious mind, and coauthor of a 126-page national bestselling book called

Jogging that came out in the late 1960s. As the long-time track coach at the University of Oregon, his résumé is remarkable: four National Collegiate Athletic Association track and field championships; in addition, he coached forty-four all-Americans and nineteen Olympic athletes. When he was away from the track, Bowerman constantly experimented with ways to remove nonessential ounces from running shoes in order to improve their performance. He said that the "ideal shoe would provide enough support for a runner during a race, but would fall apart once that runner crossed the finish line." He tried out new designs and materials for the soles, spikes and uppers.

In a 1960 *Sports Illustrated* profile of Bowerman, he was quoted as saying, "'The ordinary track shoe is covered with junk. Leather trim, tongue, laces. All unnecessary.' {The Bowerman} shoe, which he cuts and sews himself to fit the athlete, is a combination of scraps of leather, elastic and canvas which weighs only about four ounces, as against 6½ ounces for the ordinary shoe. Bowerman figures that if he cuts the weight of the shoe an ounce, he's saving the runner from lifting approximately 200 pounds in a mile race, depending upon the runner's stride."

Bowerman's collegiate runners were accustomed to his restless nature, unorthodox manner and tough love. One of those track men was an above-average middle-distance runner named Phil Knight, whose personal best for the mile was 4:10. After acquiring an MBA from Stanford, where he wrote a seminal paper, "Can Japanese Sports Shoes Do to German Sports Shoes What Japanese Cameras Did to German Cameras?" Knight traveled to Japan, where he was able to secure distribution rights to sell Onitsuka Tiger running shoes in the United States. He then entered into a handshake agreement with his former coach in 1964 to create Blue Ribbon Sports. While Knight kept his day job as an accountant, their fledging startup—which was going up against German footwear giants Puma and Adidas—sold 300 pairs of these inexpensive flat-soled sneakers in their first year, mainly to high school and college runners in the Pacific Northwest, often by showing up at track meets with a car trunk full of Tigers.

Revenue at Blue Ribbon Sports grew each year, fueled in part by a small sales team of passionate runners. Meanwhile, Bowerman's design ideas led to the creation of a new Tiger running shoe called the Cortez, which had a rippled rubber sole for traction and a dual-density foam wedge for additional cushioning support and shock absorption. The inclusion of a slight heel-raising wedge resulted from Bowerman's belief that it would help coax a runner forward and reduce the strain placed on the Achilles tendon. (Little did he or anyone know at the time that this small wedge would one day take on a massively metastasizing life all of its own and influence running shoe design for years to come.) The distinctive Tiger stripes on the sides, which first appeared on the Mexico 66 models, were there to provide midfoot reinforcement. The Cortez was released right after the 1968 Mexico Olympics. Despite going up against both Adidas and Puma and their well-entrenched sales and promotional machines, the Cortez quickly became a top-seller running sneaker in the U.S. due to Blue Ribbon's more aggressive grassroots marketing.

Phil Knight parted ways with Onitsuka and Tiger in 1971, a decision that was ultimately rooted in mutual distrust over sales territory and distribution rights. This divorce led to several years of a fiercely contested legal battle; but during this period, Knight's new company (later renamed Nike) was busy selling a somewhat similarly designed shoe, which was also called Cortez but made with lightweight nylon uppers and a suede toebox. (It debuted in early 1972). Following a 1974 U.S. district court judgment that was based on trademark infringement, Tiger was forced to change the shoe name to Corsair and pay Blue Ribbon monetary damages. Knight's swashbuckling crew in Oregon kept the Cortez name.

The Cortez is one of Nike's most iconic footwear models—and not just with runners. (It's the shoe Forrest Gump wore during his transcontinental crossings.) Retro models can be easily purchased online. It has street cred with Southern California gang members who probably feel like they are always running from the cops. In 2008, Lil Rob, a popular Mexican-American music producer and rapper, wrote a hit song called "Cortez shoes," whose lyrics include these lines: "These Cortez shoes know all the hard times that we had been through. All the crazy things we used to do just to get by walk in my shoes and you . . ."

First the wedge, then the waffle-sole. Each was born from Bowerman's fertile imagination, and together, they were largely responsible for Nike's success as a young athletic footwear company. As a descendant of pioneers who had come west on the Oregon Trail in the 1840s, Bowerman had his own eureka moment in 1971. Seeking a more ground-efficient sole that could replace common track spikes, Bowerman poured a gooey, rubber-like compound into his wife's waffle iron. He then cooked the non-edible batter. The process took several attempts to get the urethane concoction just right, by which time the waffle iron became, well, toast. But the end result was an inverse-outsole waffle-pattern of nubby spikes.

Geoff Hollister, another trackman who had run for Oregon, who was Nike's third employee, was the first person to try out the new waffle-tread shoes (Hollister would drive to local races and sell Tigers to coaches and athletes from the trunk of his car, earning a $2 commission on each pair purchased.) "When Geoff Hollister slipped on Bill's first test pair," writes Kenny Moore, "he found that the 'urethene spikes' on the balls of his feet seemed to grip almost regardless of what they touched, be it track, road, grass, or mud. In the fall, Bowerman made me a pair . . . and I too felt that they had broader applications than just the track. I was so sure they were going to let me run away from Frank Shorter in the 1971 AAU cross-country race in San Diego that I got excited and ran the first mile in 4:19." Shorter went 4:30 each and every mile and won, while a dialed-back Moore placed sixth. But Moore became a complete convert to waffle-tread running shoes, and later ran a 4:03.2 in them, "thought to be the fastest mile in a flat at that time."

The rubber studs of the waffle sole offered a forgiving springiness that was welcomed not only by world-class athletes, but also by everyday runners. The shoes, as *Time* magazine then wrote, were "grabbed by the army of weekend jocks suffering from bruised feet." And it was the waffle trainer that placed Nike on the global athletic footwear map, giving Adidas and Puma a serious run for the money—and set the stage for its unparalleled growth. Today, Nike is a publicly traded multi-billion dollar behemoth with a vast array of shoes, apparel, and products for almost all the major sports. Its Swoosh logo, created for the princely sum of $35 by a young graphic designer by the name of Carolyn Davidson, has become one of the world's most recognizable symbols. (The original Swoosh went straight across the Nike letters, making it hard to read; people often mistakenly called the shoes "Mike.")

❧

Nike was named after the Greek goddess of victory. Yet early Greek Olympic athletes competed in the nude—and *without* shoes. (One might consider this a good example of irony.) That didn't mean that everyone in ancient Greece went barefoot all the time. Except for the poor or slaves, many went about their daily business in tunics, togas, and flat-soled sandals. Sandals, however, were just one of many footwear options available to Greeks as well as other vanished civilizations. But it must be emphasized that most people went barefoot—and this was true all over the world right up to the early 1800s (and remains true in some parts of the world today).

Several thousand years before Athenians gathered in the Agora to debate politics or watch plays, shoemaking was no less critical than the spear or sharp-edged stone hunting knife in terms of shaping civilization. Without adequate footwear protection, pre-modern man would have been unable to survive the harsh winter months after migrating much further north of the temperate African plains.

In 2010, a team of archaeologists found a pair of 5,500-year-old leather shoes outside a cave in Armenia, making them the oldest leather shoes known to exist. Each shoe was made from a single piece of cowhide. A lace passed through four sets of eyelets closed its rear. In the front, fifteen pairs of eyelets were used to lace the shoe from toe to ankle. Archaeologist Ron Pinhasi, of University College Cork in Cork, Ireland, who led the research team, told the press that "the shoe is similar to a type of footwear known as 'pampooties' common in the Aran Islands, west of Ireland, up until the 1950s. In fact, enormous similarities exist between the manufacturing technique and style of this (Armenian) shoe and those found across Europe at later periods, suggesting that this type of shoe was worn for thousands of years across a large and environmentally diverse region." Scientists don't know if its owner was male or female, but these pre-modern shoes would fit a woman today wearing size 7.

Previously, the oldest leather shoe discovered in Europe or Asia belonged to a well-preserved Stone Age hunter named Otzi, also known as the "Iceman," whose frozen mummified body was found by hikers in the melting glaciers of the Italian Alps in 1991. Otzi was later carbon-dated to have been between 5,375 and 5,128 years old. He was carrying a dagger, trapping net, bow stave, and some arrows. To protect his feet from the ice and rocky terrain, Otzi wore insulating hay-lined shoes made with deer and bear leather that was held together by a lattice of coarse fiber.

Petr Hlavacek, a Czech shoe expert, painstakingly recreated a replica of Otzi's shoes, and found them practical, comfortable, and durable; in fact, he felt that they actually performed better than most modern footwear. Before Hlavacek started regularly wearing the shoes on local hikes, he and a colleague took the shoes to a hockey rink and pushed each other around the ice. They found that the tanned bearskin (cured with the animal's own brains and liver), gripped the smooth surface as if it had been made with top-quality rubber. They later sampled the shoes on a treadmill with pressure-pad sensors attached to the soles, and again both men were amazed at the positive results. The hay offered greater loft and better insulation than contemporary synthetic materials. A *New Yorker* profile of the Czech shoe savant in 2005 reported that "the shoes were so well cushioned that the body's weight was evenly distributed across the soles: the peak pressure points were half as high as in hiking boots, 75 percent lower than in sneakers, and 85 percent lower than in high heels. It is miracle." Hlavacek emphasized that "in these shoes you can practically not obtain the blisters." He later remarked to another journalist "it's like going barefoot."

The ultimate assessment of Otzi footwear took place on a three-day hike in the Alps in the late fall. Hlavacek recruited several other trekkers to join him, including Vaclav Patek, a well-known Czech climber who also designed mountain-climbing shoes. All were shod in Otzi-like shoes. "Over the next three days, they climbed more than fifteen hundred meters, across snow-covered glaciers and granite scree. They trudged through streams of melt-water barely above freezing, yet their feet felt only a momentary chill. When, periodically, Hlavacek stuck a thermometer inside the hikers' shoes, the readings hovered comfortably around seventy degrees Fahrenheit. More surprising, to a climber like Patek, was how well the shoes performed on difficult terrain. Their soles were so light and flexible, their leather so adhesive, that they could easily scale granite boulders. By the time the expedition reached Otzi's gravesite, on the tenth anniversary of his discovery, Patek had declared the boots more comfortable and capable than any he'd worn. 'There is no mountain in Europe that couldn't be conquered in these shoes,' he told Hlavacek."

Hlavacek's positive experience in the Otzis had the effect of making him an anti-modern evangelist at international shoe footwear conferences. While he acknowledged the impracticality of walking around town in smelly bear-and-hay shoes, he claimed "there don't exist other hiking shoes where you cannot obtain the blisters!" Most contemporary shoes are made with artificial materials that offer no shape memory, so the foot ends up unnaturally conforming to the rigid shoe, and not the other way around. Most dress and running shoes fall in this Procrustean category, leading to a myriad of common foot ailments such as bunions and hammertoes.

The ancient Greeks were really the first to turn shoemaking into a viable commercial enterprise. Sandals or *krepis* were usually made with a leather sole and leather thongs threading between the toes and over the instep. The rich often decorated their sandals, while Greek prostitutes wore platform sandals with advertisements etched into the sole bottoms so these messages could be read in the dirt or sand where they had walked.

The Romans followed in the conquered Greeks' footsteps regarding sandal making and footwear custom, even adopting the habit of removing one's shoes while indoors. But they introduced many more footwear options that reflected one's status and occupation. Roman law dictated types and colors of footwear available to the different classes. Generally speaking, a soft leather shoe/sandal hybrid with both open and closed toes was used for the outdoors.

Since the Roman army often had a lot of ground to cover, mostly on foot, special attention was given to a soldier's shoes. The military lace-up sandal, known as the *caligae*, had many variations, depending on terrain and weather. Most were open-toed; others enclosed the foot like a regular shoe. Short nails often extended from the outer sole for improved traction. Often socks were used for added warmth and comfort.

The Roman Mile: Do the Math

The mile holds a strong emotional and physical attachment with almost all runners. The distance acts as our training and racing baseline, whether we log miles on the track, treadmill, or road. The current number of American runners who have broken four minutes in the mile is around 350; worldwide, that number jumps to 1,200. That figure could be much higher since the mile is not run as much as the 1,500 meters (also called the "metric mile") in international competition. (In the 1,500 meters, running 3:42.22 is equivalent to going 3:59.99 in the standard mile.)

So how did the mile come into being in the first place? The word is derived from the Latin or Roman word for *mille*, or 1,000, because a mile was the distance a Roman legion could typically march in 1,000 paces (or 2,000 steps, with a pace being the distance between successive falls of the same foot). And just how fast could Roman soldiers march? They typically had to cover twenty-five miles in five hours carrying a seventy-pound backpack. A soldier's average pace would have been around eleven-and-a-half minutes-per-mile.

Milestones were erected every mile on all Roman roads after 123 B.C But according to Dr. Math on Drexel University's Math Forum website, there is some history-lingering vagueness regarding the precise length of the Roman mile. "Based on the Roman foot of 29.6 centimeters and assuming a standard pace of five Roman feet, the Roman mile would have been 1,480 meters (4,856 feet); however, the measured distance between surviving milestones of Roman roads" (a number exist in England which is about 1,000 miles from Italy) "is often closer to 1,520 meters or 5,000 feet." Oh, it gets much more complicated even for those who aced the math section on the SATs.

Since miles of varying lengths were used throughout Western Europe, in 1592, the British parliament finally settled the question by defining the statute mile to be 8 furlongs, 80 chains, 320 rods, 1,760 yards or 5,280 feet.

That was the distance that Roger Bannister covered in 1954 on the Oxford, England, track when he clocked the very first sub-four minute mile. At the time, it seemed like an impossibly heroic feat, the human equivalent of a jet smashing through the sound barrier. But the world record for the mile was 4:01.4, which was set by the Swedish runner Gunder Haag in 1945. All Bannister really had to do was whittle away 1.5 seconds over four laps, or just under 4/10ths of a second every circuit.

Bannister ran the mile in 3 minutes and 59.4 seconds. His two pacesetters had positioned him well for a 59-second last lap. By his own estimation, Bannister said afterwards that he had run 20,000 miles in eight years of ceaseless preparation for the day of reckoning.

Seven weeks later, the Australian John Landy broke Bannister's record by going 3:58. The times have dropped ever since. Hicham El Guerrouj, of Morocco, holds the world record in 3:43.13. Ironically, Bannister, arguably the most famous miler, is also the man who held the world record for the shortest period of time.

Roman footwear design and workmanship had a lasting influence long after the Empire's fall. It was not until the early Middle Ages that shoes abandoned their original usefulness and began exhibiting scant regard for the human foot. That was certainly the case with the English pikes or points (also called *poulaines*), long-snouted shoes that often extended twelve inches beyond the foot.

Historians believe that trade with Near Asia and the Orient was responsible for this new footwear trend, since it meant the arrival of new textiles, fabrics, and designs that included satin, pearls, and silk. For much of antiquity, however, the Chinese were, like the Romans, quite practical when it came to shoemaking, using animal hides, cloth, and leather thongs, except when it came to the barbaric custom of foot binding. This required first breaking the bones of a young girl's feet, then wrapping the entire foot painfully tight to prevent further growth. The practice was thought to have originated among court dancers in the tenth century. It then spread to the wealthy and later to all classes, even among the poor. Tiny, distorted female feet were considered sensuous, beautiful, erotic. The crippled feet also forced a woman to adopt an unnatural yet highly enviable gait called the lotus walk. The Communist Party finally outlawed foot binding in the late 1940s. By then, it has been estimated that as many two billion Chinese women had their feet bound.

England's King Edward III in the late fourteenth century decreed that pointed shoes (the Church considered the *poulaines* phallic and sinful) could have no more than two additional inches. But it wasn't long before another fad took hold: padded and heavily embroidered "duckbill" or "bear's claw" shoes that featured a super-wide toebox, reaching up to a foot in diameter. Since the wearer could barely walk in these clown-like shoes (the gait was more like a waddle), another English law was passed limiting the width to no more than six inches.

But shoe-design experimentation was only just getting started. Because shoes were made with expensive textiles and fabrics, they needed protection from the muck and grime of roads. Pattens were overshoes that were worn over one's good shoes, and usually consisted of a thick sole made of wood and leather straps. Not to be outdone, Italy and Spain saw the birth of wood or cork-based *chopines* with a raised platform sole that could reach as high as twenty inches. For aristocratic women, walking around in chopines was like teetering around on stilts and typically required an attendant or servant to prevent them from falling over. Because the chopines' height symbolized the wearer's social standing—the higher the shoe, the higher the status—it's easy to see why they remained popular all the way into the seventeenth century. Chopines were the nine-inch Jimmy Choo stilettos of their time.

Whereas *chopines* elevated the entire shoe sole to mega proportions, isolated elevation of the heel might have had its origin in Asia. In a 1972 article titled "Footgear—Its History, Uses and Abuses," author Steele Stewart, M.D., describes Persian figurines depicting thirteenth-century Mongol conquerors like Genghis Khan outfitted with block-heeled boots. Stewart discusses several possible scenarios that could have led to the development of the heeled boot among Mongol warriors. One possibility is that the heel allowed horsemen to better steady themselves in stirrups while using weapons during battle; another was that the heel served as a prosthesis for wounded soldiers.

Whether the heel that made its way to Europe in the sixteenth century was a result of migratory horsemen from Central Asia is still up for debate, but the heel has been an entrenched element of footwear design ever since. Along with pumps and slipper-like shoes, heeled shoes became popular in pre-revolutionary France amid the upper class and royalty, for both women as well as men (who favored low, broad footwear). Large shiny buckles, often composed of silver or gold, became another must-have fashion accessory. Stacked leather heels were used in men's boots, almost always made in black. All types of boots, from riding to walking, came to dominate footwear in the mid 1700s and all the way into the late 1800s.

One of the most significant developments in shoemaking was the introduction of automation in the early part of the nineteenth century. Until the 1840s, shoes were handmade, and the shoemaker used hand tools and a hardwood or cast-iron mold called the last that approximated the shape of a human foot. (Sandals didn't require a last since the entire foot wasn't enclosed.) Most shoe lasts were straight, meaning there was no difference between the right or left foot. Breaking in new shoes was not always a comfortable proposition. With the advent of the rolling and sewing machine, footwear could now be mass-produced. Factory-made shoes built around uniform lasts (now for each foot) became affordable and widely available. In his 1885 book, *The Art of Boot and Shoemaking*,

John Bedford Leno can barely contain his disgust over the kind of shoes coming off the assembly line. "Despite of what has been said regarding the improved form lasts have been made to assume since their manufacture became a separate industry, many of the lasts supplied to boot and shoemakers are totally unfit for use. . . . There is no recognized standard among last makers, and they differ to such an extent that it is practically impossible that all can be correct."

Unless he favored boots, the late 1800s man primarily wore one of two kinds of leather shoes—laced-up oxfords or brogues (which is a low-heeled shoe or boot). Surprisingly, men's shoe fashion has remained fairly static ever since (apart from sports shoes).

On the other hand, women's shoe designs have seemingly changed with the seasons. For a lady's footwear closet, this has been true for centuries, and it's certainly true today. Take the modest Victorian woman; she usually wore a long dress and pointed, ankle-high laced boots so that no bare leg could show. Contrast that with the 1960s when women preferred miniskirts and knee-high go-go boots. (Nancy Sinatra's number-one hit song, "These Boots Are Made for Walkin'," came out in 1966.)

Recent footwear styles for women might seem to suggest that high-heeled shoes are the norm. But according to a 2011 consumer survey conducted by *Footwear News*, "barefoot/minimalism" led the pack, followed by vintage, lightweight running shoes and espadrilles. Who knew! Yet, when celebrities like Scarlett Johansson are photographed running in Vibram FiveFingers, one can see why. Ranking near the bottom were platform shoes and stilettos.

Indian Running and Footwear

North of Laguna, two Zuni runners sped by them, going somewhere east on Indian business . . . They coursed over the sand with the fleetness of young antelope, their bodies disappearing and reappearing among the sand dunes, like the shadows that eagles cast in their strong, unhurried flight.
        —Willa Cather, from the novel *Death Comes for the Archbishop*

North America's first great long-distance runners were Indians. The Iroquois Nation, an alliance of tribes scattered throughout the northeastern region of the continent, used a communication network of specially trained runners, who typically traveled in pairs or small relay teams. These couriers would carry messages between villages along the 240-mile Iroquois Trail. For protection from small rocks and roots, the runners wore a small piece of cured animal hide such as deerskin that was stitched with sinew and perfectly conformed to their feet. These soft, flexible shoes were called "makasin," a name etymologically derived from the Algonquian word "maxkeseni." The word became known as moccasin in English when the white settlers arrived from Europe, clumsily clomping about in their heavy boots or stiff leather shoes with broad heels and buckles.

There are historical accounts by European newcomers who were astonished by how little noise the Indians would make walking or running. One report: "{The two Iroquois runners} took their way through the forest, one behind the other, in perfect silence." But few white men wore moccasins unless they were trappers or military scouts. A barbaric stigma was associated with going native.

Almost all North American tribes used moccasins. (Shoe names were different.) Many of them added decorative artwork, such as detailed beadwork and quillwork. Indians could easily tell another's tribal affiliation simply by looking at the footwear construction and design. Geography was a key determinant of style. The Plains Indians wore moccasins of hardened soles made from buffalo or deer hide because of the rocky soil. Southwest Desert Indians, such as the Hopi, Zuni, Navajo, and Apache, combined two pieces of animal hide for a thicker sole as protection from flesh-piercing thorns and cacti needles. In colder, mountainous regions, rabbit fur was used as lining. The Inuit (Eskimos) crafted calf-length, heavier-duty boots called mukluks that were made from sealskin fur and reindeer hide.

If you check the Internet, you can find several sites selling do-it-yourself moccasin kits. Large footwear companies like Minnetonka sell "moccasins," despite their having half-inch Vibram rubber soles, making a mockery (pun intended) of the original concept. A much smaller shoe outfit, Soft Star, which is based in Corvallis, Oregon, has been making moccasins for over twenty-five years. Its original RunAmoc (with a thin two-millimeter Vibram sole) might look like something Peter Pan would wear, but the shoe (and a low-ankle version) has received positive reviews from minimalist trail runners.

Foot messengers and the runner-relay system played an integral role with other Indian tribes, including the Fox, Sauk, Creek, Omaha, Kickapoo, Osage, Menominee, Pawnee, Apache, Zuni, and Hopi. Like with the Iroquois, runners connected families, clans and villages. But with the Hopi, running also served a deeper, more transcendent purpose. Footraces were held in order to strengthen social bonds and connect participants to the spirit world. Stories of past footraces were an important part of the Hopi oral tradition; they meticulously passed down from generation to generation.

Matthew Sakiestewa Gilbert, an assistant professor in American Indian Studies and History at the University of Illinois, has studied and written about Hopi footraces. He's also Hopi. The March 2010 issue of *American Quarterly*, an academic publication, published an essay by Gilbert entitled "Hopi Footraces and American Marathons, 1912–1930." He writes, "Since the beginning of Hopi time, as first evidenced in the Hopi clan migration stories, long-distance running has held a vital role in Hopi society. According to Hopi belief, the Hopitu-shinumu, or 'all people peaceful,' emerged into this fourth world, or 'fourth way of life,' from a series of three underworlds." The Hopis would have running races in the hope of appeasing their gods to bring rain to their frequently parched fields.

In time, other gods needed appeasing, but these were mortal gods— white men in neckties and straw hats, who wielded stopwatches at track meets and races where Hopis were encouraged to compete. These officials didn't care a whit about rainfall or the spirit world; they were more interested in seeing who could run farthest and fastest. And the Hopis could fly like the wind over long distances of harsh terrain. Their natural talent for running mirrored the Tarahumaras who lived much father south in the secluded mountains of northern Mexico.

Gilbert recounts what one anthropologist in the late 1800s witnessed at a running race: ". . . The Hopi runners ran barefoot and plunged into cactus and thorny bushes without the slightest hesitation. Hopi races required each clan to kick a small ball to the end of the course, and as they worked together, the Hopi runners demonstrated incredible skill, endurance, and an ability to keep the health of the entire Hopi community in mind. . . . In the kick-ball races, the Hopi Cloud gods rejoiced 'to see the Hopi youth run,' as running allowed their prayers for rain to be heard.'"

But the late 1800s was not a hopeful period for Hopis. In 1882, U.S. President Chester Arthur passed an executive order creating a reservation for the Hopi Indians, an area of land much smaller than the nearby Navajo reservation. Hopi children were forcibly shipped off to boarding schools to make them "more civilized," but running still ran deep and strong in their blood.

America's first running star of the 1900s was Louis Tewanima, a Hopi who attended the Carlisle Indian School in Pennsylvania. This was the same school that Jim Thorpe attended. (Born of mixed race ancestry in the Oklahoma territory, Thorpe had an Irish father and a mother who was part-Sac and part-Fox Indian.) Generally considered to be the country's fastest marathoner, Tewanima competed for the United States in the 1908 Olympic London Games, where he finished ninth in the marathon. Four years later, he took silver in the 10,000 meters at the 1912 Stockholm Games, where Thorpe won the decathlon. Tewanima's 10K time of 32:06.6 set a United States record that stood for fifty-two years.

Any American long-distance runner who wanted to compete in the Stockholm Games marathon needed a top-three finish in a qualifying 26.2-mile race that was held in Los Angeles. One hundred and fifty runners were invited to compete. Fifteen thousand people lined the streets to watch. As Gilbert writes, "Two Hopi runners, Guy Maktima and Philip Zeyouma, stood beside the many athletes who gathered near the start line and waited for the sound of the pistol to begin the race. The Hopis ran for the newly established cross-country team of Sherman Institute, an off-reservation Indian boarding school in Riverside, California." A reporter for the *Los Angeles Times* noted that Zeyouma wore "moccasins" that Hopi women made for him on the reservation, and a shirt that depicted the legendary "winged" (flying) snake of the Hopi.

At first the Hopi runners 'received no attention from the other athletes who 'kept their eyes on the many famous' runners in the group. During the initial two miles of the race, the Hopis positioned themselves near the front of the pack, but refrained from making a sudden advance for the lead. At the halfway point, the Hopi runners increased their pace and shortened the gap between them and the other frontrunners. "When word spread among the thousands of spectators that the 'little Hopis' had broken away from the lead group, people rushed to the finish line and waited for the runners to make their final approach." The moccasin-wearing Zeyouma won, but for some unknown reason, he later declined to compete in the Olympics.

Tewanima was a crowd-drawing attraction in a number of U.S. races, and he did not let the spectators down. In 1920, Tewanima placed first in the 20-mile Mardi Gras race in New Orleans as well as the *New York Evening Mail* modified marathon.

Among the Hopi today, Tewanima is a deeply revered name. In 1974, the Hopi Athletic Association began sponsoring the Louis Tewanima cross-country race. The Hopi reservation, with a population of 7,000 people, stages several fun runs and trail races each year. The Hopi running tradition lives on.

If most runners have little familiarity with the name Tewanima, one can blame Hollywood for neglecting to put his life on the big screen like it did with Jim Thorpe. A very non-Indian-looking Bert Lancaster played the mighty athlete in the 1951 film *Jim Thorpe—All-American*. Thorpe never received a dime from the movie. Most shameful was that Thorpe was unable to find steady work after a short-lived career playing semi-pro football and baseball. He'd occasionally appear as a film extra when a director needed someone to play an Indian chief. Adding insult to injury, B. F. Goodrich produced a line of children sports shoes called Chief Long Lance that were "endorsed" by Thorpe. (Why didn't they just call them Thorpes?) Sadly, the century's greatest all-around athlete died broke two years after the biopic was released.

Two Indians have won the Boston marathon. The first was Thomas Longboat of the Onondaga Nation in Ontario, Canada, who set a course record in 1907. Ellison Brown, a member of the Narragansett Indian tribe of Rhode Island, was the second. While known as Deerfoot among his own people because of his speed, the press gave him the nickname "Tarzan Brown" due to his muscular build. At Brown's first Boston race in 1933, his cheap canvas sneakers fell apart, and so he ran the last five miles barefoot, finishing the marathon in thirteenth place. Three years later, he won in 2:33; his second victory came in 1939 with a time of 2:28.

Another outstanding Native American runner was Billy Mills, who won the 10,000 meters at the 1964 Tokyo Olympics. A member of the Oglala Lakota Sioux Tribe and a U.S. marine, Mills's life story was biographically recreated in the 1984 movie *Running Brave*, which starred Robby Benson, another odd casting choice. (Benson, whose birth name was Robin David Segal, grew up in New York City; both his parents were Jewish.) No American has ever duplicated Mills's Olympic feat in an event that's now dominated by East Africans.

A fair question to ask is how come the Tarahumara don't compete on an international level like the Africans? The short answer is cultural. Tarahumara comes from the native word Raramuri, which means "foot runner." Their endurance running feats have been written about since the early 1900s. Two Tarahumara competed for Mexico in the 1928 Amsterdam Olympics marathon, but race officials neglected telling them beforehand that the course was "only" 26.2 miles long. Not too far off the lead, they continued running past the finish line until officials stopped them. "Too short, too short," they said afterwards.

In his 1981 book titled *Indian Runner*, author Peter Nabokov writes, "It seemed like the Tarahumara, as with other Indians, found it difficult to extract their running prowess from its cultural context and reshape it to fit the white man's criteria for competitive sports." Running on a cinder track in endless circles supposedly gave them nightmares afterwards. The crowds were another element that created individual angst. "The scrutiny of howling strangers contrasted with the support of backers and friends at home and the winding stretches of quiet mountain trails." Then there was the practical issue of footwear. "The cleated leather shoes required at Olympic meets did not conform to their splayed, bark-hard feet."

The Leadville Trail 100 is a vivid example of the cultural disorientation experienced by Tarahumara when they were thrust into a foreign running environment. In 1992, Rick Fisher, a Tucson-based wilderness guide and photographer, invited several Tarahumara to compete in the Leadville race, an ultramarathon that is held in the Colorado Rockies. Most of the course's elevation is over 10,000 feet. None of the Indians finished the 100-mile race, but the reason was not because they were under-trained.

"The problem, it turned out, was an unfamiliarity with the trail and the strange ways of the North," reported Don Kardong of *Runner's World*. "The Indians stood shyly at aid stations, waiting to be offered food. They held their flashlights pointed skyward, unaware that these 'torches' needed to be aimed forward to illuminate the treacherous trail. And so on. All five Tarahumara dropped out before the halfway point."

But the following year, the first-, second-, and fifth-place finishers were Tarahumara. The oldest, Victoriano Churro, fifty-five, won the race in just over twenty hours. At the first aid station, thirteen miles into the race, the Indian trio removed their running shoes that had been provided by Rockport, which was one of the race's main sponsors. Then each runner laced up his huaraches that he had made the previous day by using leather straps and discarded tire treads found at the Leadville landfill. The three runners covered the next eighty-seven miles in their primitive, handcrafted footwear.

The Tarahumara haven't been back to Leadville. There's no compelling reason for these bashful, reclusive people to travel to the U.S. and compete in an ultra. Ironically, their absence from the international endurance running scene has been recently overshadowed by their influence on contemporary running and minimalist footwear. *Born to Run* made them world-famous. Barefoot running has subsequently taken off. And running huaraches like Luna Sandals and Invisible Shoes (rebranded in early 2012 as Xero Shoes) have become increasingly popular.

Early Athletic Shoes

Another important development in shoe manufacturing was the use of rubber. The earliest "sport shoes" were produced by a Liverpool rubber company in the 1830s. Primarily worn by the Victorian classes, they were known as "sand shoes" or "plimsolls" because the lines formed by the rubber and canvas bond looked similar to the curving Plimsoll line on a ship's hull. The real breakthrough of incorporating rubber into footwear occurred in 1844 when the American inventor Charles Goodyear received a U.S. patent for hardened, or vulcanized rubber. (His original interest in the strange, flexible properties of natural latex gum was marked by a desire to make life preservers.) Yet it wasn't long before rubber started regularly appearing as soles for athletic shoes.

These new species of shoes, with canvas uppers and rubber soles, were often called "sneaks" in slangy homage to cat burglars and thieves because their bottoms made little noise when one was walking or running. Sneaks later colloquially morphed into the word "sneakers." When U.S. Rubber launched Keds athletic shoes 1917, they were marketed as sneakers. (See "The Story of Keds.") But the footwear manufacturing process of using rubber proved tricky, since it required a lot of trial and error. Plus the shoes often fell apart after limited wear. Hence, the preferred shoe for physical activity such as for walking, running, or playing cricket (in England) was one made entirely of leather. In fact, early spiked athletic shoes were made for cricket. As for the provenance of the first specifically made running shoe, footwear historians point to a pair owned by Lord Spencer, with a fairly reliable date of 1865. Interestingly, the Spencer running shoe looked like little more than a leather, square-toed dress brogue with spikes attached to the sole—it even had a sizable heel lift.

The mid-1800s also marked a period when footraces of various distances—walking and running—became common in England, a trend that eventually made its way to America. The sport was called pedestrianism. Exhibitions featuring professional walkers and runners going around a single track for up to several hundred miles attracted large crowds and substantial prize purses. Wagers were placed on these races. America's most famous endurance walker was Edward Weston who, in 1871, walked 400 miles in just five days around a New York City track. But by the 1880s, pedestrianism lost its luster due to claims of price-fixing and the rise of amateur athletics. The latter was an elitists' attempt to weed out the workingman, immigrants, and ethnics from what was considered a gentleman's pastime. As such, wagering on sports and prize money for professional athletes were discouraged. With its emphasis on team camaraderie and character-shaping, collegiate sports like football, rowing, and track and field became popular instead.

The 1896 Olympics, which were officially known as the Games of the First Olympiad, became the catalyst for increased interest in athletic footwear development. The Athens Games struck a popular chord, especially among Americans and the English, who valued the healthy benefits of physical culture. They took up bicycling, hiking, bodybuilding, boxing, tennis, and calisthenics with renewed vigor and passion. With regard to the sport of running, the newly-minted marathon inspired by the Athens' race became the rage—but as a spectator pastime. The first Boston Marathon (just under 25 miles) debuted one year after the Athens Games with fifteen starters. Ten runners finished. By 1902, the field nearly tripled to forty-two runners, with over 100,000 spectators lining the course. Runners wore lightweight ankle-high boots or flat shoes with leather uppers and soles.

While the Boston Marathon is the world's oldest continuous marathon, it was not the only race of its kind in the United States. There was the Dipsea, a 7.4-mile trail run on the West Coast that premiered in 1905 and was billed by the *San Francisco Examiner* as "the greatest cross-country run that was ever held in this or any other country." One hundred runners competed in the inaugural event that ended at Stinson Beach. (The Marin County race with its 688 tortuous steps at the beginning is still going strong with an always sold-out field limited to 1,500 runners.)

Towards the end of the nineteenth century, direct-sales copy for running shoes began to appear in the Sears catalog and elsewhere. "Men's English Running Shoes" in the 1895 Montgomery Ward catalog went for $2.35, and were made with "fine cordovan leather and wooden bottoms."

A British running enthusiast and shoemaker by the name of Joseph William Foster had achieved limited commercial success making running spikes for local runners. In either 1904 or 1905, he came out with the "Foster's Running Pump" that was suitable for asphalt roads, grass, and dirt. The Pump, arguably the first all-purpose running shoe, sold well and provided Foster and his sons a good living for years to come. In 1960, two of Foster's grandsons assumed ownership of the company and renamed it Reebok after the Dutch spelling for an African gazelle. Nineteen

The Story of Keds

If you were a boy growing up in the 1950s or 1960s, then you probably owned a pair of Keds. Even more likely, as soon as your pair of Keds wore out, you or your parents bought another pair of the canvas-top sneakers. Keds were popular on baseball diamonds, in backyards, and on school playgrounds all across America. The U.S. Keds logo, a blue rectangular patch on the rubber trim along the heel, was as familiar as Coca-Cola's. But not any longer. Starting in the early 1970s, the brand's popularity declined, unable to keep pace with changing consumer tastes and the marketing budgets of large athletic shoe companies such as Nike and adidas. Boys stopped wearing Keds for gym class and sports. And it wasn't too long before teenage girls started wearing them instead as a retro-chic fashion statement, along with baggy socks and colorful leggings. Keds are still worn today as casual vintage sneakers, but their place in the athletic footwear scheme of things is quite small.

The story of Keds began in 1892 when the U.S. Rubber Company started producing soft-soled croquet shoes using the patented Goodyear process of vulcanized rubber. In response to an increased demand for rubber-soled athletic shoes, U.S. Rubber and Goodyear merged to create a new sports footwear company. The original name was going to be Peds (from the Latin word meaning "foot"), but another company had already trademarked that name. So it chose Keds.

The first Keds' print ads used the term "sneakers." The ploy worked as a means of quickly garnering attention and market share. In 1949, Keds introduced a new line of sneakers called Pro-Keds, which were designed for more serious athletic performance. Its main competition was Converse and its popular Chuck Taylor All-Star basketball shoes.

In 1963, Keds began running television ads featuring a pear-shaped clown named Kedso who encouraged kids to sing this jingle: "If you want shoes with lots of pep, get Keds. For bounce and zoom in every step, get Keds." In one commercial, Kedso asked two live-action boys in black high-tops why they wore Keds. The much larger boy replied, "So I can ran faster and jump farther."

Keds also ran a series of commercials featuring Kolonel Keds who flew around in his jetpack before dropping down to the ground and telling young boys that "Keds are scientifically designed like my Bell Rocket Belt . . . with a built-in {cushioned midsole} booster pad to give you more get up and go." That so-called booster pad was less than a quarter-inch of compacted foam rubber.

As Keds began to falter as a footwear brand, it bounced around several different rubber companies. Today, Keds is owned by Collective Brands who acquired it from Stride Right.

years later, in a footwear version of the British music invasion, Reebok landed on the American shores courtesy of Paul Fireman, an enterprising U.S. sporting goods distributor whose timing was impeccable. The aerobics craze was just around the corner. In 2006, Fireman sold Reebok to adidas-Salomon for $3.8 billion and personally cashed out to the tune of $800 million. Hoping to strike footwear fire again, just five years later, Fireman acquired a minority interest in Boulder-based Newton Running for $20 million.

The Spalding Company had once dominated the American sporting landscape the way Nike now does. In 1908, Spalding came out with its all-new running shoe. The "Spalding Marathon Shoe" resembled a soldier's low-profile boot, with a gum-rubber sole and leather heel that was reinforced with rubber. And it was expensive for its time—eight dollars a pair. But sales were disappointing because the soles would partially disintegrate after just one race. By 1911, Spalding removed the gum rubber outer sole altogether and added an inner rubber sole for cushioning and comfort. But early rubber technology was no match for the demands of long-distance runners, and within two years, the Spalding shoes, now renamed "Correct Marathon Shoes," featured all-leather soles.

Marathon fever spiked right after the 1908 Olympics when an American by the name of Johnny Hayes won the gold medal in the 26.2-mile footrace after the soon-to-be-disqualified winner Dorando Pietri, of Italy, collapsed upon entering the Olympic stadium and race officials helped him make it to the finish.

Several marathons, for example, held in the New York City area, attracted elite runners and large crowds of spectators. There were also shorter races billed as "modified marathons." In May 1912, 1,300 runners ran from the Bronx to New York City Hall in a 12-mile race sponsored by the *Evening Mail*.

Public fascination with the marathon, and running in general, waned during the First World War. However, American interest in athletics reemerged during the sports-mad Roaring Twenties. Johnny Weissmuller won five gold medals in Olympic swimming and set sixty-seven world records, Bill Tilden ruled the tennis court with dapper flair, Bobby Jones tore up the golf links, Jack Dempsey stalked the prize-fighting ring with iron fists, and Babe Ruth filled up baseball stadiums with a steady barrage of home-run blasts. Economic times were prosperous for many Americans; the leisure class grew and lifestyles shifted accordingly. Self-improvement turned into a national pastime. Dale Carnegie became a household name. Diet and calorie-counting books for fashion-conscious women were instant bestsellers. Men flocked to the gym to lift weights, box, and swing wooden Indian clubs. Even the Boston marathon saw resurgent growth, though it wasn't until 1964 that the field ever had over 300 runners.

The Bunion Derby

There was one sporting event that best symbolized the athletic spirit and brio of the Twenties: a 3,400-mile transcontinental solo run that the press coined "The Bunion Derby." On March 4, 1928, 155 men, ranging in age from late teens to early sixties, left Los Angeles and headed to New York with the starry-eyed dream of winning the $25,000 first-place prize promised by the event promoter, Charles Pyle, who was one part P. T. Barnum and the other, Don King.

According to Charles Kastner's book, *Bunion Derby*, these runners represented a melting pot of first-generation immigrants, blacks, Native Americans, Midwest farm boys, former Olympic champions, and professional race walkers. It even attracted the attention of the greatest ultrarunner of his generation, a forty-four-year-old South African by the name of Arthur Newton.

The course followed U.S. Route 66 out of Los Angeles. Hundreds of thousands of spectators lined the two-lane highway. "Most of the contestants wore tracksuits," writes Kastner, "but some donned overalls, street clothes, and flannel shirts. The well-prepared had specially built running shoes with dozens of pairs in reserve, while others wore logger boots or moccasins, or in a few cases, no shoes at all." A caravan of support vehicles followed behind, carrying a portable tent city, along with cooks, physicians, nurses, massage therapists, and skilled shoe repairmen working out of the back of a "shoe hospital truck."

The daily pace set by the leaders during the first week was fast and brutal, often averaging seven minutes per mile for thirty-five or forty miles. The South African Newton smartly lagged behind in the middle or rear, maintaining a consistent speed. Two weeks into the race, the field had been halved. Foot, leg, and stomach ailments had taken their toll. The racing conditions were harsh, unforgiving—desert heat, wind, freezing rain in the mountains. Yet the remaining bunioners courageously forged ahead, willing their broken-down bodies to make it to the next town or stage, then sleeping each night "in drafty tents and learning to survive on Pyle's meager food allowance that left many scrounging for food from local citizens."

Despite winning a wind-whipped stage in Arizona, covering forty-four miles in seven hours and ten minutes, Newton was later forced to withdraw from the Derby, informing a race official, "My legs are gone. I knew that it will be impossible for me to continue." A previously strained Achilles tendon had forced him to compensate by overworking his uninjured leg.

As the Bunion brigade made its way east along Route 66—New Mexico, Texas, Oklahoma, Kansas, Missouri—a fraternal-like bond developed among the remaining sixty-four runners, many of whom had little expectation of winning even though cash prizes went ten deep. On Day sixty-three, the runners arrived in Chicago where Route 66 stopped. Thousands of spectators lined Michigan Avenue, as a sailor from New Jersey by the name of Johnny Salo won that stage. Only "another thousand miles" to New York City were left for the exhausted road warriors.

On the eighty-fourth day, a twenty-year-old Oklahoma farm boy, who was one-eighth Cherokee Indian, crossed the finish line in Manhattan with the lowest cumulative time of 573 hours. Andy Payne had averaged ten minutes per mile for 3,400 miles. That moderate pace was strictly enforced by Payne's trainer/manager who counseled the lad to "ignore the temptation to race for stage victories."

Despite all the press and hoopla, the Bunion Derby left its promoter Charlie Pyle flat broke. But the indefatigable showman was a big dreamer who somehow managed to pull off a second race the following year. This time, however, the Derby started on the East Coast.. Only eighty men competed this time, including Newton, second-place finisher Salo, and third-place finisher Peter Gavuzzi, a short steamship steward from Liverpool, England, who reportedly would smoke a pack of cigarettes during his long workouts. Payne didn't enter, choosing instead to join the entourage as a rope-twirling entertainer in the race's evening tent show.

Once again, the field dwindled quickly, but after seventy-eight days of running, it came down to a tight race between Salo and Gavuzzi, with only minutes separating the two endurance athletes. Due to some logistical confusion on the final day in Los Angeles, the Englishman lost by just two minutes and forty seconds. Even more unsettling to Gavuzzi and others was the news that Bunion promoter Pyle had run out of funds. Instead of winning a cash prize, each of the top-ten finishers received worthless promissory notes. Later that fall, the stock market crashed, the Great Depression set in, and the Bunion Derby was never held again.

If you were one of those early Boston marathoners, like the legendary Johnny Kelley, who won the race in 1935 and 1945 and finished second seven times, your banged-up feet paid the price of running two-and-a-half-hours in ill-fitting shoes. When Kelley won his first Boston race, the Spalding catalog featured just one marathon shoe that was made with low-profile leather uppers and a rubber outsole. In *The Running Shoe Book*, author Peter Cavanagh describes Kelley's constant footwear predicament: "{He} tried anything he could get his hands on which was lighter, kinder to the feet, and cheaper than the Spalding shoes. He ran races in sneakers, bowling shoes, high jump shoes." In 1992, at the age of 84, Kelley, the retired Boston Edison electrical maintenance man, who was later named "Runner of the Century" by *Runner's World*, completed his sixty-first and final Boston marathon.

But Spalding wasn't the only shoe available for runners in the 1930s and 1940s. During this period, a retired English-born shoemaker in his seventies named Samuel Ritchins felt that he could build a better footwear mousetrap for runners. So he began handcrafting lightweight running shoes called S.T.A.R. Streamlines. Their distinctive foot-stabilizing features included side lacing, a separate heel, easy-to-mend outsole, and a smoothly constructed toebox. The shoe's appeal was solidified at the 1940 Boston marathon when nine of the first eleven finishers wore Streamlines.

Meanwhile, over in Europe, two German brothers, Adi and Rudi Dassler, had started making sports shoes called Dassler in their mother's laundry room. As sales steadily increased, they eventually expanded operations to a small factory in their home town of Herzogenaurach. Prior to the start of the 1936 Berlin Olympics, they somehow persuaded Jesse Owens to wear Dassler spikes. After Owens won four gold medals at the 1936 Berlin Olympics—100 meters, 200 meters, long jump, and as a member of the 4x100 meter relay team—Dassler sports shoes became world famous. Now all coaches and trainers wanted their athletes to compete in these Teutonic track shoes. The brothers were soon selling 200,000 pairs of shoes each year before the Second World War. Then, the story of the Dassler duo turns sinister, murky and downright weird. The two brothers joined the Nazi party and began making shoes for the German army, but a deep rift developed between them when Rudolf was arrested by American forces and sent to a prisoner of war camp. He thought his brother had ratted him out. They separated as business partners in

1948, with Adi starting his own shoe company now named adidas, while Rudi created a new sports shoemaking firm that he called Ruda before later changing it to Puma. The fierce rivalry between these two brother-led companies split the Bavarian town literally in half. Herzogenaurach became known as "the town of bent necks," because local residents "would not strike a conversation with a stranger until they had first looked down at the shoes that person was wearing," observed Barbara Smit, who chronicled the history of adidas and Puma in her book *Sneaker Wars*.

Most sports in this country went on a hiatus during the Second World War, but when the U.S. troops came home, interest immediately returned and old taboos were overturned. Jackie Robinson broke baseball's color barrier with the Brooklyn Dodgers in 1947. The Olympics returned with London as the host city. Wearing his black Converse Chuck Taylor All Star high tops, Bob Cousy led the Boston Celtics to six NBA championships in the fifties. Pugilists Rocky Marciano and Sugar Ray Robinson dominated their outmatched opponents in the boxing ring.

With respect to running, the 1950s witnessed the following: a history-setting performance in the mile, continued greatness by an Olympic long-distance champion, and a footwear footnote. Let's begin chronologically.

The 1951 Boston Marathon winner was Shigeki Tanaka, nineteen, of Japan, a survivor of the Hiroshima bombing, who crossed the finish line in 2:27:45 while wearing "tabi" or split-toe running shoes. A two-year-old Kobe footwear company called Onitsuka, which was named after its founder and is best known today as ASICS, had developed the tabi running shoe by modeling it after the traditional Japanese sandal (*geta*) that had a strap between the big and second toe. For some reason, Onitsuka stopped making tabi-style running shoes several years later, and when it started exporting running shoes to England and the U.S. in 1960, the athletic footwear featured a standard shoe design. So why didn't the split-toe running shoe become popular? Was the West suspicious or uncertain about the quality of "made-in-Japan" products? Of course, the tabi running shoe appeared odd and unfamiliar to non-Japanese. But the tabi sneaker seemed a lot less peculiar than Vibram FiveFingers when they were introduced in 2005.

Emil Zatopek is widely recognized as one of the greatest runners of the twentieth century. The Czech runner bettered his 1948 Oympics showing (gold in 10,000 meters and silver in 5,000 meters) with his famous "hat trick in Helsinki" at the 1956 games. Tacked onto Zatopek's victories in the 10,000 and 5,000 meters was an astonishing marathon win—a race he had never run before. In the space of six years, from 1948 to 1954, the former Bata shoe factory worker won a total of thirty-eight consecutive 10,000 meter races, while also setting eighteen world records in various distances ranging from the 5K to 30K. Known as the "bouncing Czech" because his running style was exceptionally awkward, with his head spastically moving to and fro like a bobble doll, Zatopek significantly raised the bar when it came to training. Along with long runs to build up stamina and endurance, he incorporated interval sprints and slow-running recoveries. He'd often train in his heavy combat boots. He felt that it was an efficient way to enhance leg strength.

More conventional in his training methods but equally committed to being the world's best, Roger Bannister only started running as a freshman at Oxford University in England. He had never worn running spikes previously or run on a track. His workouts were light, consisting of only three weekly half-hour sessions, but he showed early promise in running a mile in 1947 in 4:24.6. After a disappointing showing at the 1952 Olympics in the 1,500 meters, Bannister, who was also studying to be a doctor, considered giving up running. But he fixated on a new goal: to become the first man to run a mile in under four minutes. He ramped up his workouts.

Training was one thing. Shoes another. He sought out a Wimbledon-based shoemaker who hand-fashioned track spikes with uppers that were made from soft, lightweight kangaroo skin. The spikes were extra long, as menacing as piranha's teeth.

On May 6, 1954, the day of reckoning arrived. A prestigious British amateur track meet was being held in Oxford. Bannister's morning began in his research laboratory where he further sharpened the spikes. Years later, he told a British newspaper, "I remember a medical colleague scoffing, 'you don't think that's going to make a difference do you, old boy?' He didn't understand I was looking for anything which might shave 0.01 seconds off my time."

Bannister's meticulous preparation paid off. Before a crowd of 3,000 wildly cheering spectators, he broke 4 minutes. The new mile record made newspaper headlines across the globe.

When the 1950's snapped shut, not much had changed in running footwear since the pre-war era. Although Bannister and Zatopek captured everyone's hearts and minds, the affection stopped there and didn't extend to the public's feet. This was due in large part to market demand. Running was still an esoteric sport, practiced by a tiny elite of self-motivated, highly trained athletes who competed for personal glory, high schools, colleges, amateur track clubs, or their country during the quadrennial Olympics. Footwear companies saw little need or sales opportunity that would warrant retooling their factory assembly lines to begin mass-producing running sneakers. The recreational runner simply didn't exist. But the sixties changed all of that—in a totally unexpected way that forever altered the sport of running.

CHAPTER 5

⟡

The Recreational Runner

My suspicion is that the effects of running are not extraordinary at all, but quite ordinary. As runners, I think we reach directly back along the endless chain of history.
—JAMES W. FIXX, AUTHOR OF *THE COMPLETE BOOK OF RUNNING*

The sixties began, curiously enough, with an anti-shoe bias among a distinguished roster of champion runners. We all know about the unshod Abebe Bikila whose bare feet flew over the cobblestones en route to winning the marathon at the 1960 Rome Olympics. (The Ethiopian runner wasn't the first marathoner to go barefoot in the Olympics; that honor belongs to South African Tswana runner Len Taunyane, who finished ninth at the St. Louis Games in 1904.) Fewer of us are probably familiar with the serial accomplishments of Herb Elliott, a talented Australian middle-distance runner who appeared twice on the cover of *Sports Illustrated*, in 1958 and 1960, each time running barefoot!

Elliott held the world record in the mile (3:54); and at the Rome Olympic Games, he won the gold medal in the 1,500 meters and bettered his own world record with a time of 3:35.6. He trained under the tutelage of his iconoclastic coach, Percy Cerutty, who embraced a mind-body, holistic approach to training that was centered around barefoot runs on the beach and sand dunes, discussing poetry and philosophy for mental stimulation, avoidance of wheat flour, and no water or liquids during meals. It also helped that Elliott possessed a graceful, natural running stride. From 1957 to 1961, Elliott was the preeminent middle-distance runner in the world. During this four-year stretch, he *never* lost a 1,500-meter or mile race.

Known as "Europe's Barefoot Champion," England's Bruce Tulloh won the European 5,000 meters championship in 1962 by racing unshod on the cinder track. Tulloh had started running barefoot three years earlier because he was convinced that shoes were slowing him down. In short order and without shoes cramping his style, Tulloh won his first British amateur title barefoot and continued racing and setting U.K. records, including the two miles in 8:34, until he retired from competition in 1967. Two years later, he ran across the U.S. in sixty-four days—but he wore shoes due to his uncertainty about road conditions. Tulloh, seventy-six, who lives in Marlborough, England, went on to coach many top British middle-distance runners, authored several books on running, including a popular one called *Running is Easy*. He even spent a short spell in the early 1970s in Mexico's Copper Canyon with the Tarahumara Indians and, like others who have had that opportunity, was amazed by how far and effortlessly they ran in their huaraches.

In 1961, Tulloh, who later became a biology instructor at a small British college for twenty years, was briefly placed under the microscope by a famous medical researcher interested in barefoot running. Dr. Griffith Pugh, who achieved fame as medical leader of the 1953 Everest climbing team, tested Tulloh on the track. In a 2011 interview with *Running Times*, Tulloh described the process: "Dr. Pugh had me run repetition miles, to compare the effect of bare feet, shoes, and shoes with added weight. He collected breath samples. It showed a straight-line relationship between weight of shoes and oxygen cost. At sub-5:00 mile pace, the gain in efficiency with bare feet is 1 percent, which means a 100 meter advantage in 10,000 meters. In actual racing, I found another advantage is that you can accelerate more quickly."

Barefoot racing was also popular among other elite British runners, such as Ron Hill, who ran barefoot when he took second in the International Cross-Country Championship in 1964. The following year, the shoeless endurance athlete won the Beverley (England) Marathon, in 2:26:33. At the Mexico Olympics, he placed seventh in the 10,000 meters—again *without* shoes. Hill also told *Running Times*, "I was going to run the marathon at the 1972 Munich Olympics barefoot, but the Germans laid new stone chippings on parts of the course."

In the United States, Dale Story, a junior at Oregon State, won the 1961 NCAA cross-country championship by running barefoot. In a recent interview with an Oregonian newspaper, he reminisced, "People laughed at me. There were acorns on the course. Those guys thought I was absolutely crazy. They said, 'Man, you're going to hurt your feet.' Didn't bother me at all."

Given the fact that these highly accomplished runners—Bikila, Elliot, Tulloh, Hill, Story—had achieved success *without* shoes, then why didn't more of their contemporaries take up barefoot running? One likely reason might have had to do with perception and habit. Perhaps there was something retrograde, an anti-modern reversal of the *natural* order of things, about barefoot running that made it seem far too primitive to have any real appeal for almost all westernized runners at the time. Or maybe it was due to practical concerns like having one's unprotected feet encounter broken glass, sharp objects, or unwanted debris. These are all legitimate considerations that continue to resonate today among runners.

But in the early 1960s, there was something else standing directly in the path of barefoot is best. Quality running shoes designed specifically for road racing and training had finally begun to appear—not in mass quantities by any means, but in limited numbers. Runners looking for that competitive edge were drawn to Tiger Cubs that were manufactured by Japanese-based Onitsuka. The lightweight Tigers had flat-bottom rubber soles, were easy on the feet, and held up pretty well. They could be purchased via mail order for the discerning few. Demand was still quite small because running was very much a fringe sport attracting only the diehards.

"The 1960s," says runner Hal Higdon, who went onto become a well-known author and contributing editor for *Runner's World*, "was a decade both dark with despair and bright with hope, an era when the Boston Marathon attracted only a few hundred starters, most of them capable of breaking three hours. Nineteen fifty-nine was the year I ran my first Boston. We were a scurvy lot, the 150 of us who showed up in Hopkinton, our deeds largely unheralded." At least, this small, nearly invisible group of malnourished American and British long-distance runners now had the option of running in decent shoes.

In 1960, a Boston custom footwear and arch-support company called New Balance came out with a non-cleat running shoe called the "Trackster" that featured a rippled-rubber sole. It was also available in different widths. William Riley, an English immigrant, founded new Balance in 1906. He initially made only arch supports; but in the mid-1920s, he began designing running shoes for a Boston running club known as the Boston Brown Bag Harriers. The shoe's success led to additional sales, and by 1941, New Balance was creating custom-made shoes for baseball, basketball, tennis and boxing.

Apart from its unique sole and a name that suggested it was aimed for track runners, the Trackster looked a lot like a two-toned golf shoe. It was sold primarily to local college cross-country and track teams at MIT, Tufts, and Boston University. Ad copy for the Trackster promised "natural foot action—the result of design based on orthopedic principles." Its patented "Ripple Sole" guaranteed that a runner could "lengthen his stride, reduce fatigue, improve traction, prevent stone bruises and shin splints."

A small crew of workers produced up to thirty pairs per day of the Tracksters, a number that held constant until 1972, when under new ownership, New Balance ramped up its operations to meet the intense demand of a new running boom that had begun to sweep across the nation; and Boston was its epicenter. Sales skyrocketed for New Balance, which is today a global footwear giant (one-quarter of its shoes are still made in the U.S.).

So just how and why did that explosion in running occur in the first place? What or who lit the fuse? Health crazes had gripped the national imagination before, like in the twenties, only to later fizzle. What made this era profoundly different? And why did running stick around, becoming more and more popular, experiencing nearly fifty years of sustained growth? According to a published report by *Running USA*, over 500,000 runners finished a marathon in 2010. The half-marathon number is even more staggering: 1.4 million finishers. How did running make the quantum leap from scurvy to mainstream, and what did this mean for runners and the constantly changing footwear landscape?

During the fifties, America had morphed into a sedentary society of flaboholics. Cars replaced walking. The television became a fixture in households. Most men expressed their lackadaisical commitment to fitness by mowing the lawn in their nine-to-five work shoes or playing golf on the weekends. For stay-at-home women, exercise was mainly limited to following easy-workout evangelists like Jack LaLanne on their black-and-white sets.

It was rare for a man to lace up his athletic shoes and go for a short run even in his own neighborhood. (For women, it was even more of a rarity, or as the trailblazing Kathrine Switzer, who was the first official woman to run in the Boston Marathon, remarked, "Back then, sweating in public was very unfeminine.") When the late George Sheehan, a cardiologist in the small town of Rumson, New Jersey, took up running in the early sixties at age forty-five, he felt like such a complete misfit that he went out of his way to cloak his embarrassment. Years later, his son Andrew wrote of his father, who was a top miler at Manhattan College in the early 1940s: "Initially, he took pains to hide the fact that he was running at all. Running in public would have been viewed as subversive in a town such as ours—perhaps in any town. Thus he began his running in the privacy of our backyard."

It took Sheehan twenty-six loops to complete a mile in his backyard. That came to just under 70 yards per lap. The circuit must have gotten boring in no time, or perhaps he felt more daring, because Sheehan soon started running along a river road during his office lunch break. In the winter, he wore long johns and a ski mask to ward off the cold.

"I found running," Sheehan later said, "and that made it the best year of my life. I was in middle-age melancholia. I had to pull the emergency cord and get off the train. Before I ran, I was getting bombed every weekend. I didn't smoke because I was too cheap."

Five years later, Sheehan clocked a 4:47 mile, which marked the first sub-five-minute time ever by a fifty-year-old. But his real passion occurred away from the oval track as he began competing in road races. He ran in twenty-one consecutive Boston Marathons.

Sheehan chronicled his experiences and personal observations in a local newspaper, and from that column, he went onto become the medical editor for *Runner's World* and author of eight bestselling books on running. Through his writings and well-attended lectures held at running clubs throughout the U.S, he became widely known as the philosopher of the recreational runner, motivating millions to get off the couch and take to the streets. "Listen to your body," he exhorted his rapt listeners.

About 2,500 miles away, in Eugene, Oregon, another late-in-life recreational running evangelist was busy delivering a similar message. A trip
to New Zealand in 1962 with his University of Oregon track squad had
opened Bill Bowerman's eyes to running's limitless possibilities for the
common person. He had just turned fifty, and was overweight and out
of shape; but the hard-driven, hyper-competitive coach discovered within the space of two weeks that slow-paced running could improve one's
heart-health, shed extra pounds, and gradually build endurance. He fell
in love with the simple, unencumbered pleasure and healthy benefits of
running for fitness instead of for speed. Slow running even had its own
name: jogging.

Bowerman's epiphany came as a direct result of his fortuitous interaction with another well-known running coach: New Zealand's Arthur
Lydiard, a formerly overweight rugby player whose "radical" training
methods of combining long, slow distance runs with intense workouts
seemed to reap great dividends for himself and his stable of top athletes.
One runner, in particular, became an international track superstar. Peter Snell took Gold in the 800 meters at the 1960 Rome Olympics.
In 1962, Snell set the world record in the mile; and two years later in
Tokyo, he scored an Olympics twofer: winning both the 800 and 1,500
meters.

Two other Lydiard runners won distance medals in Rome. Back home
in New Zealand, Lydiard became an instant national hero. And he wisely
used that fame to his advantage. Jeff Galloway explains how in his book,
Galloway's Book on Running: "After the Olympics, he was frequently invited to speak to groups of sedentary men and women in their thirties, forties, and beyond. The people he talked to began to sense that they could
run gently and improve their physical condition. Running not only could
take off the weight, but could be fun. Lydiard transformed the public's
image of running from an intense, tedious, painful activity into a social,
civilized component of the active New Zealand lifestyle. He got them out
of their chairs and onto the roads in the early '60s, and the underground
running movement began."

Shortly after his return to Oregon, a slimmer and more energized
Bowerman (he lost ten pounds) started a jogging class at the college track
for Eugene residents. On the first day, only several people showed up.
When a rumor spread that *Life* magazine was sending a photographer

to the cinder track, over a thousand townsfolk showed up for the third class. What happened next was actually a good thing. Bowerman was alarmed that many of those who wanted to become runners were in horrible shape. The book *Swoosh* paints a vivid picture of the unfolding scene and its aftermath:

> *Bowerman took one look at the crowd and got scared. . . . They were expecting him to turn them into sub-four-minute milers overnight. But they were just townspeople—businessmen and housewives who hadn't done a lick of exercise in ten years. He was afraid that if he got them up and running that someone was going to have a heart attack right out there on the track. Deferring to his better judgment, he climbed up on the steps and told them all to go home.*

Never one to abandon a good idea or personal project, Bowerman decided to hold his jogging class again several months later, but this time everyone had to first pass a physical supervised by a local internist by the name of Dr. Waldo Harris.

The class's most eager students were about two-dozen women who showed up in "capris and loafers or jeans and tennis shoes. These women jogged in quilted nylon car coats with pleated plastic rain caps on their heads against the early morning drizzle, or curlers topped with pincurl bonnets with froufrou ruffles. . . . The Cinderellas, the women joggers called themselves" were there to get in shape. The exercise routine was simple and straightforward: "twenty steps walking, twenty steps jogging, twenty steps walking, twenty steps jogging." Everyone followed the Lydiard philosophy: "Train, don't strain."

In 1966, Bowerman and Harris wanted to broaden the message that jogging was fun, healthy and easy to do, so they created a twenty-page pamphlet that went for fifty cents and was available at YMCAs nationwide. About 2,000 copies were distributed this way. Jogging's big breakthrough came the following year with the publication of their 126-page book, *Jogging: A Physical Fitness Program for All Ages,* with a local writer James Shea helping out.

Over 1,000,000 copies were eventually sold. Jogging became a household word and activity. It's simple to see why. The book made jogging accessible for all Americans, whether they were fit or fat, young or old, husband or wife. Here's an early passage from the book:

Jogging is different from most popular physical fitness programs. Unlike weight lifting, isometric exercises and calisthenics with their emphasis on muscle building, jogging works to improve the heart, lungs, and circulatory system. Other body muscles are exercised as well, but the great benefit comes from improving the way the heart and lungs work. After all, when you are past 30, bulging biceps and pleasing pectorals may boost your ego, but your life and health depend upon how fit your heart and lungs are.

The first half of the book lays out the basic principles of jogging, explaining why it's good for the body and then offering tips on form (posture, breathing, foot strike), choosing when or where to run, and goal-setting. Sprinkled throughout these pages are photos of everyday joggers of all ages, including several women wearing full-length car coats and plastic rain hats. The second half of the book presents three 12-week training plans that are based on one's level of overall health, fitness level, and weight. Each plan combines jogging with some walking for the duration of the three-month period. Plan A, for example, starts with only doing a half-mile workout three times a week; at the end of the training period, the jogger is doing one and one-half miles. Plan C, which is for "men and women in better than average physical condition" tops out at four or five miles three times a week. All three plans include some walking or stretching on off or "rest" days.

What was the average speed of these joggers who were hoping to reach the goals set forth in one of the three plans? The book has a pace chart with suggested speeds, ranging from 15-minute miles to 7-minute miles. The authors state, "Faster than 7 minutes per mile is a run, not a jog."

They also provide the following invitation to readers, yet one can detect a slight hint of worry in their tone:

Jogging is a simple type of exercise, requiring no highly developed skills. The great appeal is that it is so handy. Almost anyone can do it anywhere. Our concern is to keep it simple, not let it become hidden in some mystique full of rules and paraphernalia.

Well, running today often seems to be taken over by rules and paraphernalia, especially when it comes to footwear (or lack thereof). But it's extremely doubtful that Bowerman, despite his uncanny visionary gifts, could have seen the future on these twin fronts. No one is that clair-voyant. And despite his involvement with three-year-old Blue Ribbon Sports, whose annual sales were just over $80,000, and his continuing effort to design a better Tiger running shoe, the highly principled Bower-man deliberately went out of his way in *Jogging* not to recommend any particular running shoe. Tiger gets no mention whatsoever.

Then what did Bowerman suggest that joggers wear on their feet? The full extent of his recommendation is found in just four short paragraphs on page 33:

The Shoes Should Fit

If your feet are going to carry you to fitness, they must be treated well. Your shoes are an important item. A number of firms specializing in sporting goods make shoes especially for track and long distance running. You may purchase a pair or get by nicely with what you have at home.

As you grow older, your foot needs an extra cushion.

In general, shoes should be sturdy with rubber, crepe, ripple or neolite sole. Preferably, the shoe you wear for gardening, working in the shop or around the house will do just fine.

Sneakers and tennis shoes are all right if they are the heavy variety. The fashionable, lightweight "tennies" that school girls and some housewives wear won't hold up or provide the comfort you require for jogging.

This is not to say that Bowerman was shoe agnostic for elite runners, like the national caliber speedsters he coached at Oregon. They need-ed the lightest, most optimal footwear. For his steeplechase runners, he made track shoes by hand that featured nylon net uppers. He then sug-gested to Onitsuka that it might want to manufacture road-suitable Tiger running shoes with an upper made of nylon fabric instead of leather. In 1967, Onitsuka came out with the very first running shoes using nylon, the Tiger Marathon.

Nylon was a game-changer for the fledgling running footwear market. Shoes were lighter and dried faster. The second game-changer occurred shortly afterwards: the slight heel wedge, another Bowerman creation that came as a result of his growing concern that all of these new joggers were getting injured. In fact, he had personally conducted research in Eugene with a small team, including a local orthopedic surgeon, to investigate this new exercise malady. Luckily, no one was suffering heart attacks from jogging. Instead, these new fitness aficionados were suffering from foot and leg injuries—shin splints, Achilles tendonitis, knee pain. Bowerman realized that maybe it was the running shoe itself that caused these unanticipated problems to arise. Then what was intrinsically wrong with the running shoe? It had a flat sole. And all these newly minted joggers lacked the proper foot and leg strength that more experienced runners had developed over time. Consequently, too much strain was being applied to the Achilles tendon, setting in motion other biomechanical problems in the feet and legs. So Bowerman recommended to Onitusuka that they begin making shoes with a half-inch raised heel. Bowerman believed that this wedge would not only lessen the repetitive stress impact of the jogger's feet hitting the ground, but also nudge him or her forward, almost like getting a slight, invisible push from behind. The Japanese company heeded his words, though to Bowerman's dismay, the heel of the new Cortez Tiger was raised only three-eighths of an inch.

The era of the flat-soled running shoe was gradually coming to an end. It would take another forty years before the tide would begin to change in the opposite direction, when thick tread, large-heeled shoes started ceding some of their market share back to flat-soled running shoes. For commercial reasons, the phrase "flat sole" was replaced by a newer, hipper term—"barefoot." When the Nike Free debuted in 2007, it was billed euphemistically as "the first barefoot running shoe." There was still a noticeable heel-to-toe drop, but the non-rigid, flexing, barefoot-style sole was a definite departure from the recent past.

⌘

Along with Sheehan and Bowerman, another middle-aged individual played a significant role in the growth of running in the late sixties. Dr. Kenneth Cooper was the author of 1968 bestselling book *Aerobics* that turbo-charged the fitness revolution and running boom. He encouraged millions of readers to walk or run at least four times a week, while maintaining that the harder you physically pushed yourself, the healthier you'd become.

To this trio of running evangelists, we must add another person: 1972 Olympic marathon champion Frank Shorter. Almost all running historians and followers of the sport mark his victory in Munich, and later, his marathon silver in the 1976 Montreal Games, as the single most influential driving force behind the sudden rise in recreational running and marathon participation in the U.S. He inspired the masses to become runners. Let's briefly use the Boston Marathon (which another legendary runner, Bill Rodgers, dominated in the seventies, winning four times), as a case study here. In 1970, 1,174 runners, who had a qualifying time of 4 hours, competed in the Boston race; the field size dipped down by about 100 the following year, but edged back up by 200 the subsequent year. And for the next several years, Boston increased by 300 or 400 runners. By 1977, the field reached 3,040, and men (ages nineteen to thirty-nine) needed a 3:00 qualifying time; for all women, it was 3:20. By 1981, the field had more than doubled to 6,881, with the qualifying time dropping to 2:50 for men. When prize money wasn't offered to the professional runners, the numbers began to decrease, but then once money was on the table, the field grew to 9,416. On the hundredth running in 1996, 38,708 runners started the centennial race. From 2003 to the present, the field has averaged between 20,000 and 25,000 each year (43 percent of racers in 2011 were women), and that's because of stringent qualifying standards. Otherwise, the total number of runners would be much higher, easily approaching that of say, the New York Marathon, which went from 127 competitors in its first year in 1970 to its current field of around 35,000 racers.

It's difficult to fully know what exactly makes one determined to run in a marathon, but thirty or so years ago, the marathon runner was primarily white and male, and likely emboldened to take up the sport after reading Jim Fixx's *The Complete Book of Running*. A decade after *Aerobics* became a bestseller, this book by a middle-aged Vermont runner who used to be overweight, sedentary, and a heavy smoker, motivated countless couch potatoes to take up running for the first time. It too sold over a million copies. The book's red cover—Fixx's lean muscular legs, red shorts, and a pair of red , thin ripple-soled Tigers—became iconoclastic and highly recognizable. (For its April 2012 cover story on minimalism, *Running Times* paid direct homage to Fixx's book by photographing elite masters runner and natural running advocate Dr. Mark Cucuzzella in a somewhat similar gait pose, albeit taken outdoors and with Mark wearing blue shorts and classic blue Tigers.)

Footwear Arms Race

As the running boom of the seventies swelled the ranks of joggers and recreational runners into the millions, athletic footwear companies like Nike experienced phenomenal growth, as did ASICS, New Balance, and adidas. They answered increased consumer demand with built-up shoes offering the latest in comfort, cushioning, and support. It turned into an R&D arms race for feet. New technologies, materials, and design features were constantly being refined and developed.

The decade began with Tiger racing and training flats as the top choice for runners. According to a survey of 800 runners conducted by *Runner's World* in 1970, seventy percent of them wore Tigers, followed by adidas at 43 percent, the short-lived Lydiard shoe at 10 percent, and New Balance at 8 percent. (Runners owned more than one brand.) In terms of individual shoe rankings, the Tiger Cortez was number one, then the adidas Olympia and Tiger Boston.

By 1973, the newly formed Nike, despite being involved in a litigious battle with Tiger, became a serious player, garnering 20 percent of the training flat market. Adidas fought back by introducing a heel counter. And in the following year, Brooks Shoe Company came up with a special foamlike polymer compound called EVA (ethylene vinyl acetate) that was lighter and a better shock absorber than rubber. The new Brooks Villanova used EVA for its midsole and heel wedge. In a short time, EVA became a fixture in most running shoes for the burgeoning recreational running market.

When *Runner's World* conducted its annual shoe survey in 1977, the top twenty-five shoes, according to Peter Cavanagh's *The Running Shoe Book*, "had a raised 'Achilles tendon protector' at the heel and all but four had flared heels {for rearfoot control}. It was clear that many manufacturers were moving toward a consensus of design." The number one shoe in 1977 was the Brooks Vantage, which was considered revolutionary because it incorporated a "varus wedge, which created and elevation on the inside of the heel compared to the outside." Cavanagh points out that the rationale for the varus wedge was that "many running injuries stem from excessive pronation which this wedge helps prevent."

The next major innovation in running shoe design was the air-filled midsole. Nike was the first with its air shoe called Tailwind in 1979; the tubes arrayed within the midsole were filled with pressurized freon gas.

More cushioning was the holy grail for runners. The Tailwind was also the first running shoe priced at $50. Many runners loved this high-tech shoe despite its unstable rearfoot and the tendency for the air to leak from the midsole.

When the 1970s had come to a close, the New York City Marathon had expanded to 12,000 runners and there were shoes for almost every kind of runner. The 1980 *Runner's World* shoe survey, according to Cavanagh, "tested 178 models of shoes compared to the 15 that had been available in 1967. The number of shoes for women had increased dramatically with sixty training and ten racing shoes available. Not only were the numbers increasing, but so was the quality."

And yet, the injury rates among runners, as we have pointed out in previous chapters, had not diminished. This baffling trend only fueled a desire among running shoe companies to spend even more money in research and development to perfect a shoe that would reduce injuries. Was this goal even realistic?

A fascinating passage titled "The Past and the Future" in Cavanagh's book, which was published in 1980, neatly sums up the history of the running shoe.

> *If anyone thought that the evolution of running shoes was a short and simple matter, that idea must have now been abandoned. The journey of almost 10,000 years has been long and involved. What is so intriguing about tracing the history is that it mirrors the growth of something that has become completely assimilated into our way of life. By a strange twist of economics, sociology, and psychology running has become a vehicle for fitness, relaxation, and for the expression of personal well-being.*
>
> *To think that we are at the end of the evolutionary process rather than at an intermediate way station would be foolish. The changes and improvements over the next ten years will probably dwarf all that has gone before. Technology has entered the running shoe equation to stay. We shall see better shoes, safer shoes, and faster shoes.*

Cavanagh was both right and wrong in his assessment. Footwear changes in the 1980s did indeed "dwarf all that has come before." For example, adidas introduced the Micro Pacer in 1986 that had an actual microprocessor sewn into the tongue of the left shoe; an LCD display would show the runner's speed, distance, and caloric expenditure. It was the first running shoe to retail for $100. One year after its annual sales revenue reached $1 billion, Nike, in 1986, came out with its Air Max marvel that had see-through windows in the front and rear of the soles. The idea was to allow the wearer to witness the air-cushion technology. The Reebok Pump that debuted in 1989 featured a pumping unit also sewn in the tongue. The runner could then adjust the fit of the shoe to snugly and comfortable encase the foot.

Were any of these shoes or the hundreds of models from the other footwear companies that annually flooded the marketplace "better, safer, and faster" than their predecessors? Once again, if safer was defined by fewer injuries, then the answer was "no." A lot more money and R&D resources were thrown at the problem. Running shoes of the following two decades continued to flaunt space-agey designs, featherweight materials, and shock-absorbing motion-control features.

What Is a Minimalist Shoe?

"For run specialty retailers, less was definitely more in 2011. Without question, minimalist/barefoot shoes are the biggest story of the year." So read the opening paragraph of a feature article, "Minimalist 2.0—The Next Generation of Running Shoes Take Hold," in the January/February 2012 issue of the shoe trade magazine *Footwear Insight*. Citing figures from Leisure Trends Group's Run Specialty RetailTRAK, the article reported that "minimalist footwear sales totaled $45 million through the end of October 2011, up 153 percent from $18 million during the same period in 2010. Meanwhile, traditional running shoes struggle to maintain sales and share with sales trending down across the first 10 months of 2011 . . . At the beginning of 2011, minimalist shoes accounted for about five percent of pairs moving through run specialty. By the end of October, most major footwear brands including New Balance, Nike, Saucony and Brooks launched new or expanded minimalist product lines, propelling minimalist shoes to 11 percent of total pairs sold for the month."

Considering the fact that sales of minimalist running shoes were just under $5 million in 2008 (less than 1 percent of total pairs of running shoes sold), the rate of sales growth over the past three years is indeed remarkable.

Yet it's to be expected that with any new footwear trend, a lack of consensus among manufacturers can often muddy the waters for runners. Minimalist shoes are a prime example of this happening. Nothing is to stop a company from marketing a shoe as minimalist, when in fact, it might appear anything but when compared to other brands.

Clarification is clearly needed about what minimalist is, or isn't. Put simply, a minimalist shoe is one that more closely approximates the barefoot running condition. Based on this, we offer the following criteria to help determine whether a minimalist running shoe should be labeled as such:

1. Absence of a thick, overbuilt heel-crash pad like that found in a majority of conventional running shoes.
2. Minimal height differential between the sole under the heel and the sole under the forefoot. This downward slope in the sole from heel to forefoot is also known as the drop. Most conventional running shoes have a drop of 10-14mm, whereas minimalist shoes have a drop that is considerably lower (The most minimal shoes have a completely level sole—no differential at all. This characteristic is often referred to as "zero drop").
3. Thin sole overall, regardless of heel-forefoot drop. The foot should be able to feel the ground.
4. A flexible sole so the foot bends with the shoe, no matter the running surface—dirt, asphalt, grass, rocky trails.
5. Minimal structure in the upper portion of the shoe—a layer of lightweight fabric/mesh is sufficient.
6. The shoe should be lightweight—less than 10 oz per shoe is a reasonable benchmark, though many minimalist shoes weigh far less.
7. The footbed should be relatively flat and contain little cushioning or arch support.
8. The toebox should be roomy and non-constricting and allow free movement of the toes.

Which takes us to the present, whereby the "evolutionary process" is even more uncertain and up for grabs when it comes to the future of running shoes. The barefoot-lifestyle and minimalist movement, represented by new footwear companies like Altra Running, Newton Running, Vibram FiveFingers, and VivoBarefoot, as well as an ample selection of models from major shoe players like Merrell, Brooks, and Saucony, is gaining obvious traction, steadily increasing market share and public visibility. This movement has shaken up the running industry, and nowadays it's not uncommon to see runners in motion-control shoes standing next to runners in rubber-soled foot-gloves at the starting line of a race.

What will the future hold? Will the minimalist movement be a passing fad? Or perhaps *less* shoe is better than *more* shoe? The jury is still out regarding whether minimalism is here to stay, or if it's even safe and appropriate for certain kinds of injury-prone runners. Who knows what running shoes will look like in five or ten years. Yet the positive outcome of this back-to-basics movement is that more options are available for runners, and it has caused them to re-evaluate and be more open-minded in their thinking about how to choose a shoe. In the end, it will be up to runners themselves to decide which shoes they ultimately like or dislike. After all, they're the ones who vote with their feet.

CHAPTER 6

⁓✞⁓

Pronate Nation

*I believe in keeping running simple and, in regard to shoes, that
would mean no gimmicks, unnecessary cushioning, etc.*

—Bill Rodgers

*I was a bit apprehensive about going to a specialty running store for
the first time back in the summer of 2007. At the time I didn't yet
consider myself to be a "real" runner, and all of my shoes were typically purchased online or in sporting goods stores largely on the basis of
pricing and appearance (cheap and cool-looking meant good!). I vividly remember walking into the store. The fit young female employee
asked me if I was training for a race. "Training" was a foreign word
to me at the time. Running was just exercise, a way to keep my weight
down, and shoes were just shoes. But I was training for a 4-mile race,
so I said yes, and we proceeded onward with the shoe fitting. When
I told her about my aches and pains, particularly the soreness in my
knees and shins, she took one look at my shoes and asked if I ran on
roads or trails. My response ("roads") was apparently not the right one
in her eyes. It pegged me as a beginning runner, or so I thought. I was
tempted to leave. However, her response that I was wearing incorrect
shoes for my running needs made me realize that at least I was in the
right place if I was going to get serious about the sport.*

She asked me to take off my shoes and run across the carpeted store in my socks. She watched intently from behind, and after a few laps back and forth she asked an older guy who had emerged from the stock room what he thought. They agreed that I was a moderate overpronator, and that I should probably opt for a pair of stability shoes. After determining my shoe size, she disappeared into the back room, where I could see stacks of shoe boxes piled high on shelves. She soon emerged with three pairs of shoes: Nike Air Structure Tri-ax, Brooks Adrenaline, and Saucony Guide. I tried on all three, and was shocked when she suggested that I take each for a short run around the block. No shoe store salesperson had ever suggested that I should actually do a test run in the shoes I was going to buy! Weren't they worried that I was going to scuff up the soles?

The Brooks Adrenalines felt too firm, and as a new runner I wasn't really all that familiar with the brand so I crossed them off as a viable option. The Nike and Saucony shoes both felt great on my feet—both were plush and pillowy—but the Nike's fiery red highlights caught my eye, and I liked that they had that familiar little swoosh on the side. I opted to buy them, and for the next two years I was hooked on stability shoes. I didn't dare buy anything else, because the expert at the store had told me that they were what my "moderately pronating" feet needed. The last thing I wanted was an injury that would derail my fledgling running career. Little did I know at the time just how little evidence there was to support my initial running shoe prescription . . . —PML

❧

Let's say that you've decided to embrace your inner persistence hunter and feel reborn as a runner. In a sport that requires very little in the way of equipment, perhaps the only essential piece of gear that you'll need is a good pair of shoes. As the preceding chapters have shown, shoe design has changed dramatically over the years, and the running shoe has gone from little more than a simple leather foot covering to a complex mix of synthetic fabrics, foams, and technological add-ons that are supposed to protect a runner from injury and maximize his or her performance. Furthermore, instead of having a shoemaker construct a customized shoe based off measurements taken from his or her own feet, the typical runner buys mass-produced shoes from a relatively small number of manufacturers that are typically designed to fit an "average" foot. Unfortunately, your foot shape may not fit the "average," and determining which technologies are beneficial and which are merely gimmicks can be challenging. Given these difficulties, how do you go about buying your first pair?

If you're like most people, your first thought might be to head out to the local discount store, shopping mall, or sporting goods chain store and choose the one that looks and feels the best. As soon as you enter the store, you are immediately faced with what Christopher McDougall has so aptly referred to as the "Bewildering Wall of Shoes." The shoes are brightly colored, plushly cushioned, and openly flaunt the various technological features housed within—often with little windows in the sole that allow the customer to see what kind of ultra-high-tech cushioning material is locked inside. As you scan the display stretched out in front of you, each individual shoe neatly occupying its own small, rectangular perch, you begin the process of deciding which one is worthy of taking up residence on your foot. Will it be the ASICS model with the gel pod in the sole and the shimmering gold overlays, or maybe the neon yellow Nikes with the quartet of coiled springs under the heel? It's a tough decision, and apart from appearance and externally visible technology, there's little information available to help you make your decision.

What should you do?

Well, you could simply go by price—the most expensive shoe surely is the highest quality and will provide the best protection, right? Conversely, those cheap shoes in the bargain bin will probably guarantee pain and suffering. You say to yourself, "There's no way I'm going to entrust my feet to their shoddy protection!" If you're not comfortable going it alone, you might decide to ask a clerk for some advice. Unfortunately, if you're at the local mall or one of those "big box" outlets that sells athletic shoes for just about any type of sport imaginable, you're probably not going to get much in the way of meaningful help. First off, these stores rarely stock a wide variety of shoe types, and most of what you will see are probably thick heeled, heavily cushioned shoes from just a few of the major manufacturers. Virtually all of the shoes that are on display are variants on a common theme that customers are used to and have come to expect.

Furthermore, the salesperson at a generalist store is just as likely to be a college-kid working a part-time job as they are someone who actually has extensive experience fitting a runner for a proper shoe. In many cases you may be dealing with someone who doesn't even run. If you really want helpful advice regarding shoes, you stand a better chance of getting it if you go somewhere that caters specifically to runners—you should head to a specialty running store.

Specialty running shops differ from typical sporting goods stores in that they (should) have knowledgeable staff who are actual runners—that alone is a major plus. However, even in a specialty store you are at the mercy of the bias of the individual salesperson that is there to help you choose the right pair of shoes. Some of these employees might be open-minded and highly experienced, while others might not. They might simply be following the script handed to them by the footwear brand representatives (furthermore, they might working under incentive programs offered by manufacturers to push certain shoes). Others might be strictly following a store fitting policy, regardless of whether that policy has any scientific support for its efficacy in ensuring that a runner is going to be placed in a shoe that will help prevent him or her from getting hurt.

What you will often find at a specialty running shop is that the shoes are typically neatly grouped into three major categories: neutral, stability/support, and motion control. How do you know which category you belong to? That would be the role of the store clerk, manager, or owner. One of them might watch you run across the store or on a treadmill, or if the store is high-tech, you might get filmed, and in the end you will usually be diagnosed as an overpronator (mild, moderate, or severe), a normal pronator, or an underpronator (supinator). (We'll define and discuss these terms in much greater detail in just a bit.) Alternatively, they might examine or measure your foot in some way to assess your arch height. Some shops might even have fancy pressure sensitive pads that you stand on so a computer can analyze your foot, after which it spits out a few shoe recommendations; such is the seductive power and allure of technology! How could a machine be wrong? Not knowing any better, you assume that all of this high-tech poking and prodding will result in the knowledgeable salesperson providing you with the shoe that was made just perfectly for your foot.

One way or another, the goal of each of these tests is to assign you to a shoe from one of the aforementioned categories—high-arched under-pronators and normal pronators get neutral shoes (sometimes referred to as cushioning shoes), mild to moderate overpronators are placed in stability/support shoes, and severe overpronators with flat feet are placed in motion-control shoes. These categories are not necessarily fixed, and there can be a bit of overlap. For example, some fitting guides suggest that normal pronators would be fine in a neutral or a mild stability shoe. Once your "needs" have been determined, the clerk then brings you a selection of shoes from the appropriate category, you try them on, and you choose the one that feels best (ideally on a short test run). You are comforted by the expert advice that you received, and you walk out the door with your new pair of shoes, visions of a trimmer waistline or a new personal best time in your next race dancing around in your head.

While most shoe store employees are genuinely interested in finding the best shoe for each customer, too often what happens is that their rec-ommendation is driven more by the bottom line than by a runner's actual needs. Retail shops are in the business of selling shoes and related gear, and though the clerk working the floor may have the best of intentions, shoe-fitting philosophies are sometimes set by the parent company that owns the store (especially if it's a chain), and the employees are supposed to follow certain guidelines. Given this, it might be instructive to take a more in-depth look at the fitting process inside a specialty running store. What follows is a representative firsthand account of the fitting process from a former sales manager (who asked to remain anonymous) at a large, national specialty running chain:

> If you've never been fit before, I'd complete an interview process with you re-garding any injuries (past or present), typical training terrain, training goals, current running shoes (I'd take a look at the wear pattern if you brought them in) and ask you if you've worn any orthotics or over-the-counter inserts before. For example, let's say you are a new runner and have been running in a $50 neutral shoe you bought at a shopping mall store based on looks. I let you know that our shoes, unlike the cheap, low-quality pair currently on your feet, have the latest technology and that you will notice a huge difference just in standing in them, let alone running in them.
>
> Next we move on to the foot observation. I look at your feet while you are sitting and don't notice anything odd, and I tell you that. Next I have you

stand and watch to see if your arch flattens out. Let's say that it does. Next is the walk test. I have you walk back and forth barefoot, and listen to hear if your footfalls are loud or soft. I observe whether you are rolling in, or pushing off excessively. I have you stand with your back to me so I can look at your heels and Achilles tendon. I notice that they are bowed toward the inside, which indicates that you are an overpronator.

I take measurements on the Brannock device, first seated then standing. I let you know that from a seated position to a standing position your arch lengthens one full size on the left and a half-size on the right foot. I pull out the Superfeet insoles and foot model to show you how the midtarsal joint "unlocking" lengthens your arches, and I show you on the foot model how the Superfeet insoles help control the unlocking. I explain to you that I will be choosing a shoe with medially posted support built in to help guide the foot to a more central line by controlling your overpronation. I have you try on a pair of Balega socks and you are impressed by the comfort and technology.

I go to the stockroom and choose three pairs of shoes with varying degrees of support. Since I consider you to be a moderate overpronator, I grab the Asics 2160s, Brooks Adrenaline's, and Saucony Omni's. I insert the green Superfeet to see if you can tolerate the support. You like the feel so I watch you run, first in the 2160's with green Superfeet. If the stability level is good, meaning you look like you are not rolling in and you are coming through the center of the foot and it feels great then I'd sell you that combo.

This fitting process seems reasonable, helpful, and practical. Most new runners would be impressed by the level of attention they'd get at a specialty running shop—far more than they would have gotten at a "big box" store. However, it's clear from this description that the process revolves around selling technology that will supposedly "correct" a runner's stride, with the implicit assumption being that this will minimize injury risk. The underlying premise is that many runners are inherently broken in some way, and that a special kind of shoe is needed to allow them to run without getting hurt. There's nothing like the specter of injury to get a runner to open the wallet and shell out the big bucks for an expensive new pair of shoes! Our sales manager agrees:

The complete fitting process is about selling what will appear to make running easier in the new or injured runner's eyes. In fact, this fitting process is due for a reevaluation. I see feet and runners all day long and honestly the runners most injured in the shop on a regular basis are the ones in the most expensive shoes with the latest and greatest technology. Something is not right. My reason for saying this is not to criticize my employer, but to help other runners. It pains me to see runners missing out on their target race. I've seen new runners run in old cheap 'big box' shoes then get fit at our store only to end up injured in their new insole/shoe combo. I recently told a runner to go back to his cheap old shoes and see how he felt. Pain gone. I was so glad that the owner fit him and not me, but I often think I could be actually hurting the runner rather than helping him/her.

I've been working at the store for one year, and after finishing my training period, I was the top salesperson every month. I was eventually promoted to lead sales manager. I'm not saying that out of pride but only because I know the fitting process in and out. I train the staff, and I can sell it. It's not brain surgery—it's about baffling the customer with shoe, sock, insole and apparel technology. Our individual sales ratios are based off the number of shoes, insoles, socks, and apparel sold per month. We don't receive a commission or bonus, but we are to maintain all of our sales within a particular percentage. After a year of seeing the side of the shoe business that I didn't want to know about, I'm currently looking for employment elsewhere.

Our clerk's experience is not unique. Another former specialty running store manager with many years of experience had this to say: "I have been in workshops with owners and managers of other running companies who refer to insoles as 'lunch money.' The margins are great and it's an easy sell. This is a common selling point by sales reps of insert companies." The question once again springs up—are we being sold what we really need, or what will make the most money for the store. One can only hope that it's not the latter.

The shoe-fitting process just outlined, or with some variation, is standard practice at many specialty running shoe stores (for a different take on shoe fitting, see sidebar on "Finding the Right Pair of Running Shoes" by Dr. Mark Cucuzzella). It is also the basic practice advocated by most running shoe companies, as evidenced by the fact that virtually all of them classify their shoes neatly into one of the pronation-control categories. For example, in its online shoe fit guide (as of February 2012), ASICS advocates first determining arch height, and provides footprint diagrams to which one can compare their own print using a test like the "wet-test." The wet-test is a simple procedure in which you wet the sole of your bare foot and stand on an absorbent surface like dry concrete or a paper bag. The resulting wet imprint of your foot will reveal something about your arch height. If no distinct arch is visible, you have flat feet. If there is a distinct dry area under the inner side of the arch region of your foot with a complete wet band adjacent to it on the outer side, you have normal arches. And finally, if the outer wet band is separated in the middle by a dry area, or if the wet band is very narrow, you have high arches. Your arch height can then be translated into the appropriate pronation-control category. According to the ASICS shoe fit guide, a high arched foot is said to be an under-pronated foot, and a ". . . runner with under-pronating feet is more likely to experience shock transmission through the lower legs." People with normal arched feet "typically experience minimal biomechanical problems," and people with low-arched, flat feet "tend to have over-pronating feet, which generally result in poor natural shock absorption." Based on the category determined, a runner would then choose either a cushioning (neutral) shoe, a structured cushioning (stability) shoe, or a maximum support (motion control) shoe.

The pronation-control model or paradigm is so ubiquitous and has such a primary place in the shoe-fitting process that one would think that its usage is supported by mountains of clinical and scientific data. The entire shoe-fitting process treats shoes largely as corrective devices after all, with the ultimate goal being to shift all runners into a "neutral" gait by correcting for either too much or too little pronation. What's more, runners often become so tied to their initial pronation control designation that many fear even the thought of trying a shoe outside of their assigned category—quite honestly, they're locked in for life. Belief in the accuracy of the fitting process can be so strong that even some chronically injured runners can be hesitant to change, despite the fact that the style of shoe they have been using for years has not resolved their problems (or, perhaps, might even be causing them). One would therefore hope that the initial in-store assignment is made with great care and on the basis of a strong foundation of clinical and scientific evidence. Sadly, in thinking this, one would be quite wrong.

Finding the Right Pair of Running Shoes

Dr. Mark Cucuzzella is a family physician and the owner of the nation's first minimalist shoe store, Two Rivers Treads, in Shepherdstown, West Virginia, which opened in the spring of 2010. A top masters runner, who at the age of forty-four won the 2011 Air Force Marathon outright, Mark is also the executive director and co-founder of the Natural Running Center. He shares his experience, insight, and wisdom about pronation, proper fit, and how to find a "running shoe" that best works for you.

When customers enter our store, questions always arise about pronation. Many of them have been labeled in the past as pronators by well-meaning employees at other running stores. Some claim that they have been classified as supinators. All they really want is shoes that fit, and that will help them to run injury-free. Yet the process of determining which shoe will best meet their needs is not something so simple as watching them walk or jog ten steps across the store floor. This kind of evaluation certainly won't help the runner find the right shoe.

So the first thing we do with these customers is have a conversation. We explain what pronation is. Then, we discuss the shoe-fitting process. We don't rush through this either. Every runner is unique. Some will need shoes with greater or lesser support and mobility control, depending on his or her foot strength.

Pronation is a normal function in the gait cycle, just like bending the knee or extending the hip. Pronation control can be achieved with your foot (ideally), with a shoe/insert (maybe), or both. Maximum pronation actually occurs when your heel is off the ground, so the foot's role in this process is critical.

Let's start with the foot itself, a remarkable engineering feat as described by Leonardo DaVinci: twenty-eight bones, multiple arches, and accompanying muscles and ligaments that move dynamically to balance, stabilize, and propel one forward. Children running barefoot naturally feel the ground and their muscles work reflexively to provide pronation control. Runners (with or without shoes) who have strong feet have the ability to control this motion just fine. The foot works best when it receives sensory information on where it's landing, and a firm surface is best for feedback. Overly soft shoes delay the feedback. Remember that a runner's foot is on the ground for only a few fractions of a second, so the pronation control must be immediate and strong.

Spending a lifetime in stiff, overly cushioned, and supportive shoes has diminished natural pronation control for most modern-day runners. The shoe has done some or all of the work for them. To see for yourself, try balancing on the ball of one foot. Can you hold the position for a second? Ten seconds? Thirty seconds? Can you pop off the ground with springy recoil while jumping rope? If you are having difficulty, then you may need to take certain measures if you want to transition to more natural pronation control and run in a true minimalist shoe.

Why is natural pronation control better? The foot is the magic spring that adds elastic recoil to our stride. This is free energy. When the foot is constricted by being made to "move" within a rigid shoe, it cannot work well as a spring and you need to apply more muscle force to the stride. More muscle use results in greater fatigue and less efficient running.

My recommendation to all runners is to make a gradual transition if you want to strengthen your feet. Do plenty of walking barefoot and in minimalist shoes. Start your transition to running slowly and remember that your muscles, tendons, ligaments, and bones are adapting and do not have the capacity for the added load yet. Do supplemental foot strengthening throughout the day. Stand on one foot, balance on the ball, walk barefoot in the house and outdoors when you can. This can only help your running. You may have a little soreness like with any new training. Tissues are lengthening and strengthening. Extreme soreness means you are progressing too quickly and asking the tissues to do too much too soon.

Proper Fit Explained

Two years before I opened Two Rivers Treads, I had completely rethought how a shoe should fit. It involves much more than just picking a size and sticking with it. Sizes and fit vary from shoe to shoe, and our feet can change size and shape over time. For example, I have started running many more true barefoot miles over the last year and my foot has greatly increased in thickness—I now need to consider this change when choosing a shoe.

At our store, we defy old-school thinking about sizing and narrow-shaped, ill-fitting conventional shoes. Improper shoe sizing and shape are the primary cause of ingrown toenails, bunions, corns, hammer toes, and hallux valgus. Shoes that don't fit your feet correctly can also lead to muscular imbalances in the body, leading to foot, knee, and hip injuries.

A proper fit accommodates the natural expansion of the foot upon ground contact. Excess waste is eliminated, along with everything that inhibits your foot's natural motion. Your foot is free to move and work the way nature intended it to; the way of its own barefoot motion. Call it toe-wiggle freedom. We educate on how to safely and gradually make this transition.

Yet, with sizing, most get it wrong. First, abandon the notion that you have a shoe size. Instead you have a foot size. Shoes are made all over the world and apply different shapes and standards. If you measure your foot while seated with a traditional measuring tool like a Brannock device and base your size on that you will likely be off by one to two sizes in a running or hiking shoe. Increasing one full shoe size is equivalent to adding only ⅓ an inch to the length of the shoe. Also critically important is that the Brannock device measures the widest part of the shoe at the ball. Infants and habitually barefoot individuals have feet that are widest at the ends of the toes, not the ball of the foot—this is the natural alignment of the human foot, and shoes should respect this.

Here's why many people are wearing shoes that are too small:

- When a load is applied to a foot by running or with a pack weight your foot will spread in length by up to half an inch.
- You need at least ⅛ inch or more of space in the heel and toe to allow space for a sock.
- You want ⅓ to ½ an inch of space in front of your big toe to allow room for loading and splay.
- Your foot will increase in width by 15 percent due to splay under load.
- Your foot is widest at the toes, and unfortunately most shoes are not shaped this way.

Tips on sizing:
- Do not assume that you are the same size in every shoe.
- Take your time and try several shoes on. Go run in them. Do not try them on while sitting.
- Always try both shoes on. If your feet are slightly different in size then fit the larger foot.
- Take the removable insole out of the shoe and see how your foot fits against the insole as a template. Is there room at the toes or does you foot spill over the insole? If there is no room to spare or if your foot spills over this shoe will not fit comfortably.
- Keep going one half-size up until the shoes are obviously too big.
- Try on shoes at the end of the day when feet are most flattened and swollen.
- Try shoes on with the type of sock you will wear for activity.

- For women, you may fit better in a men's shoe for width.
- Do not lace the shoes up tight. Allow spread in the midfoot and forefoot.
- Go up onto the ball of the foot. Can you put your index finger between your heel and the back of the shoe? If not, the shoe is likely too small.
- Consider not using the soft insole. This takes up space in the shoe and can interfere with ground feel.
- Walk on a firm surface when trying shoes on, not a carpeted one.
- If you are a runner you must run in the shoe. What feels nice and soft when walking is the opposite of what you need when running. Look for firmer base to allow for better sensory input and to facilitate stabilization.

Children's Shoes:

What children wear growing up has a strong influence on foot structure and function when they are adults. Given this, selection of healthy footwear for children is critical. You should select proper shoes for your children based on the following:

- Ultra-thin soles to allow adequate sensory perception, proper neuromuscular activation in the entire kinetic chain, and to complement the body's natural ability to absorb ground reaction forces.
- Low, flat to the ground profile—shoes should not have a slope from heel to forefoot.
- The materials should be soft and supple, thereby allowing natural foot function. The shoe should bend easily at the toe joints—this is where a foot is designed to bend to lock the arch on takeoff.
- The toebox should be wide enough to allow natural toe spread. Foot support is created by the natural arch of the foot with the great toe helping to stabilize the arch. When the great toe is pushed in toward the second toe (a common design flaw in many shoes which come to a tapered point), this stability is compromised. The foot produces the most leverage when the toes are straight and aligned with the metatarsals. A child's foot is widest at the ends of the toes (as should an adult's be if they have been in proper shoes or barefoot).
- A single piece midsole/outsole allowing protection on unnatural surfaces (concrete, asphalt) and natural rough surfaces (rock, trail) while allowing sensory perception and natural dissipation of ground reaction forces.
- Upper material should be soft, breathable, and washable.
- Discourage the use of thick, heavy socks as these can constrict the foot and interfere with sensory perception.

The Problem with Pronation Control

You are a pronator. Yes, you read that correctly. Interestingly enough, you are also a supinator. How is that possible? Aren't they opposites? How can one be both? Let's see why.

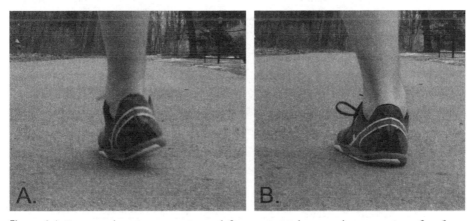

Figure 6-1. Images showing a supinated foot at initial ground contact in a forefoot strike (**A.**) and a pronated foot slightly later in stance (**B.**).

Initial ground contact in running is almost universally made somewhere on the outer margin of the foot, with the foot in a supinated position (see Figure 6-1A). Similarly, after the foot makes first contact with the ground, we all pronate. The foot begins to roll inward, everting slightly, and the arch compresses (see Figure 6-1B). Following pronation, as the foot continues through its gait, supination once again occurs. This results in the foot turning slightly outward then changing from a flexible foot to becoming rigid so that it can propel the foot and push off from the ground. During this phase the foot inverts slightly, and the arches become higher, thus enabling the foot to properly roll over the big toe.

Here's the important point though—pronation is completely normal. It's a motion that occurs in every step in every healthy foot. Pronation creates the situation in which the arch of the foot can compress, thereby stretching tissues like the plantar fascia, which store elastic energy and return it upon liftoff (like stretching and releasing a rubber band). From an anatomical perspective, movement in pronation occurs at the subtalar joint between the talus (ankle bone) and calcaneus (heel bone) located just below it, and as the foot pronates the joints of the midfoot unlock, allowing the foot to become more flexible. This helps the foot adapt to the surface, especially on uneven terrain. This, in turn, also allows the arches to compress and absorb shock. However, because the talus is also coupled above to the tibia and fibula (lower leg bones) at the ankle joint, inward rolling of the foot can also lead to internal rotation of the lower leg, which causes a twisting motion at the knee—hence the suspected link between overpronation and overuse injuries of the knee.

Because runners have long been conditioned by shoe-marketing tactics and advertising to fear pronation above all else, once they are "diagnosed" as falling into one of the pronation categories—overpronator, neutral, or supinator/underpronator—they tend to stick with shoes recommended for that category indefinitely. They are hesitant to experiment out of fear that they might injure themselves if they run in a shoe that doesn't provide the "appropriate" level of support.

Runners place a lot of faith in stability and motion control shoes to protect them from injuries resulting from the dreaded pronation of their feet. What would you say, however, if you found out that there were no data from clinical trials that have supported the use of such shoes in injury prevention? What if the tests employed by the salesperson at the shoe shop weren't very good at determining your pronation "category" to begin with? Even more startling, what if the amount that you pronate wasn't even strongly related to the likelihood that you might get injured? Scientific research has been accumulating that suggests that it may be time to reconsider the pronation-control paradigm.

In 2011, a remarkable paper titled "The effect of three different levels of footwear stability on pain outcomes in women runners: a randomised control trial" was published by Michael Ryan (then at the University of British Columbia) and colleagues in the *British Journal of Sports Medicine*. One of the coauthors of this study, Gordon Valiant, works for the Nike Sports Research Laboratory, and Nike provided footwear and funding for the study. Keep this in mind as we go through the results—the study was supported by Nike, the biggest sports shoe manufacturer in the world, and they allowed it to be published. In their introduction the authors state the following surprising detail: ". . . despite over twenty years of stability elements being incorporated in running footwear there is, as yet, no established clinically based evidence for their provision." Shocking, isn't it—despite twenty plus years of use, we have no data showing that pronation control elements in shoes are accomplishing anything of value for runners in relation to injury prevention. The study then goes on to point out that "Motion control running footwear has yet to be proven to prevent running-related injuries." Huh? Aren't these the shoes assigned to those who have the greatest risk of succumbing to an injury caused by excessive pronation? But there is no evidence or proof that they actually work to prevent those injuries? So the big question is why has the athletic footwear industry been so long wedded to a shoe-design and fitting model that has never been proven to actually work?

Given the lack of data on efficacy of pronation-control devices in running shoes for injury prevention in runners, Ryan and his colleagues decided to put the paradigm to the test. They designed a study whose goal was to determine how female runners assigned to the three categories of footwear based on their foot posture index would fare in terms of pain and injury experienced while training for a half marathon (note: foot posture index is an indirect way of determining pronation through various measures taken from the foot and ankle).

A total of one hundred and five women were classified as either neutral (fifty-one women), pronated (thirty-six women), or highly pronated (eighteen women). Now here's the really interesting part. In a shoe store, the neutral women would be assigned a neutral shoe, the pronated women a stability shoe, and the highly pronated women a motion control shoe—got it? In the study, however, the researchers took each of the three groups of women (neutral, pronated, and highly pronated), and broke them into sub-groups so that one-third would get a neutral shoe (Nike Pegasus), one third would get a stability shoe (Nike Structure Triax), and the final third would get a motion control shoe (Nike Nucleus). This was done for each of the pronation groupings, so that there would be some women in each pronation category wearing each type of shoe (i.e., many of them wearing the "incorrect" shoe for their foot).

The women in the study were then sent off to take part in a thirteen-week training program to prepare for a half-marathon to be run in Vancouver, British Columbia. Estimated weekly training volumes started around twenty kilometers and rose to a peak of about forty to forty-five kilometers. Over the course of the training program, the researchers recorded the number of missed workouts due to injury by each runner, and collected reports of pain at rest, during daily living, and following runs. Ultimately, only eighty-one of the women wound up completing the study (for a variety of reasons, twenty-four women dropped out).

The results showed the following:

1. 32 percent of the women missed training days due to pain over the course of the study. Another way to think of this is that there was an injury incidence of 32 percent in this population of runners, which is in line with other studies on running injuries.
2. Motion control shoes "resulted in both a greater number of injured runners and missed training days than the other two shoe categories." In other words, motion control shoes faired very poorly all-around.
3. Every runner in the highly pronated group who wore a motion control shoe reported an injury. In other words, all runners (yes, all of them . . . 100 percent!) who were supposed to be wearing a motion control shoe based on their degree of pronation got injured. The sample was small, but this is simply astonishing. In fact, highly pronated runners actually fared better in neutral shoes!
4. Neutral runners experienced greater pain during or after runs when wearing neutral shoes than they did when wearing stability shoes. Although the authors point out that the difference may not be clinically significant, it is once again amazing that neutral runners fared better with a shoe that would not have been "prescribed" for them in a shoe store based on their degree of pronation.
5. Pronated runners experienced more pain during or after runs if wearing a stability shoe than if wearing a neutral shoe. Again, they did better wearing the "wrong" shoe for their feet.

So what can we conclude from these findings? Motion-control shoes offered little benefit to the runners in the study, and in fact were more likely to cause pain and injury than any of the other shoe types. The fact that every single severe overpronator experienced an injury in her motion control shoes demands further investigation. In the absence of other evidence, why should anybody wear them for preventing a running injury? The authors themselves conclude, "This study is unable to provide support for the convention that highly pronated runners should wear motion control shoes."

Second, this study showed that neutral runners did better in stability shoes, and pronated runners did better in neutral shoes. Try to make sense of that finding! This is a complete reversal of what would be expected based on the current pronation-control model. This rather startling result calls into question the manufacturer practice of classifying shoes based on degree of pronation control, and it also raises serious questions about the fitting process employed by many shoe stores—should they really be placing runners in shoes based on their degree of pronation?

Ryan's study offered this rather frank assessment of the status quo: "Current conventions for assigning stability categories for women's running shoes do not appear appropriate based on the risk of experiencing pain when training for a half marathon. The findings of this study suggest that our current approach of prescribing in-shoe pronation control systems on the basis of foot type is overly simplistic and potentially injurious." This doesn't instill much confidence in the current system, does it?

By allowing publication of a study that openly states that there is no clinical data showing that shoes designed to control pronation do anything to prevent injuries, Nike took a great risk. It's comparable to a pharmaceutical company selling a drug for over twenty years that has never been shown clinically to be of any benefit to a patient who supposedly needs it. It makes one wonder if the whole pronation-control shoe paradigm is nothing more than a giant marketing gimmick whose goal is to scare consumers into buying shoes based on fear of injury. It's a time-honored marketing tactic—convince consumers of a need, and provide a product that supposedly fulfills it. In this case, the need is a neutral gait in order to reduce injury risk, and the products are the shoes that promise to correct gait to meet the need. Furthermore, in the absence of evidence showing that running shoes either do or don't reduce injury risk (or maybe even increase it), why stop making something that continues to sell and has come to be expected by consumers?

Conspiracy theories aside, the more likely scenario is that the pronation-control paradigm has simply become accepted as dogma by almost everyone, from runners, to shoe store employees, to running magazines, to shoe designers. And we would be remiss if we did not point out that the system does sometimes work—many pronated runners do just fine in stability shoes, and many underpronating runners do just fine in cushioning shoes (even some of those in Ryan's study). The problem is that Ryan's study showed that the odds of these individuals avoiding discomfort were better if they were assigned the "wrong shoe for their foot," and it is thus difficult to predict who will benefit from a given shoe and who will not.

If this were the only study showing results like this, it could be argued that it was simply an outlier, and that more work needs to be done. But, Ryan's study was not the only one that had looked at the connection between prescribing shoes based on an indirect measure of pronation and injury outcomes. Two years earlier, Joseph Knapik, an epidemiologist for the U.S. Army Public Health Command at the Aberdeen Proving Ground in Maryland, published a study with military colleagues in the *Journal of Strength and Conditioning Research* that investigated whether assigning shoes based on plantar shape (arch height) could reduce injury rates among soldiers entering Basic Combat Training at Fort Jackson, South Carolina. Their goal was to determine whether the practice of assigning shoes based upon arch height reduced injuries relative to providing all recruits a similar type of shoe.

Knapik and his colleagues examined the feet of over 3,000 recruits and categorized them as having either low, normal, or high arches. Approximately half of the recruits were then assigned to a control group and given a stability shoe regardless of their arch type, and the other half were allowed to choose an appropriate shoe for their arch type from a selection offered at the base post exchange or PX. The recruits then completed a nine-week basic training program, and injury reports were obtained from the Defense Medical Surveillance System. Results of the experiment showed that injury rates were essentially identical for the two groups—risk of injury was the same no matter whether the recruit was assigned a stability shoe, even if this was the wrong shoe for their foot, or whether they were assigned the shoe that standard practice indicated was the appropriate shoe for their arch type (and by proxy, level of pronation). In fact, the only group that showed any significantly elevated injury risk were the high-arched runners who were assigned a cushioning shoe, which most shoe fitting guides would deem to be the appropriate shoe for their foot!

Knapik and his colleagues conducted similar studies on both Marine Corps (over 1,000 individuals) and Air Force recruits (over 2,500 individuals), with largely similar results. No significant differences in injury risk were observed between the stability shoe only group and the group that went through the tailored, arch-height based fitting process. In other words, low arched recruits did just as well in stability shoes as they did in motion control, and high arched runners did just as well in stability shoes as they did in neutral cushioned trainers. In fact, the overall trend gleaned from the three military studies indicated that assigning the "correct" shoe based on arch height generally resulted in a slightly increased injury risk, though statistical differences were non-significant.

In a 2010 article on the *New York Times Well* blog, health and fitness reporter Gretchen Reynolds asked Dr. Bruce Jones, who is manager of the Injury Prevention Program for the United States Army's Public Health Command and coauthor on the military studies, what he thought about the results. "You can't simply look at foot type as a basis for buying a running shoe," said Jones. "The widespread belief that flat-

Arch Height and Injury Risk

Though many studies exist that have associated variation in arch height with certain types of running injuries, patterns are not always consistent or clear, and contradictory data are present. A study published in *Clinical Biomechanics* in 2001 by Dorsey Williams and colleagues examined arch structure and injury patterns in runners. They state that "there does not appear to be a clear relationship between arch structure and injury pattern" and furthermore that "it has been difficult to establish a relationship between a single structural deviation and a specific injury." Based upon the results of their study, they suggested that perhaps only individuals presenting with extremes of arch height deviation might experience increased injury risk.

There is also debate regarding the relationship between arch height and degree of pronation. For example, Benno Nigg, a well-known expert on running biomechanics from the University of Calgary, published a study in the *Journal of Biomechanics* back in 1993 that showed that arch height does not influence the maximum degree of eversion/pronation during running. However, he did find that when higher arched runners do pronate, they transfer a greater amount of this movement into internal rotation of the knee, which may be linked to increased risk of knee injury. Regardless, given that arch height and pronation do not seem to be strongly linked, it is somewhat surprising that the wet footprint or higher tech versions of the same approach continue to be touted as an effective means to assess pronation control needs when it comes to choosing a running shoe.

footed, overpronating runners need motion-control shoes and that high-arched, underpronating runners will benefit from well-cushioned pairs is quite simply, {Jones} adds, 'a myth.'"

So, after two decades of assigning shoes based largely on pronation control without any clinical evidence to support the practice, there are now four studies that all show the same thing: when using static measurements of the foot as an indicator of pronation, this common practice doesn't provide, on average, any real tangible benefit over simply assigning every runner a stability shoe. In fact, assigning shoes based upon arch height or other indirect measures of pronation may actually increase the likelihood of pain and injury in some cases, and some runners do better wearing the "wrong" shoes for their feet!

It's worth considering the possibility that the results of Ryan and Knapik's shoe and injury studies were skewed by the methods used to match shoes to subjects. In other words, maybe the shoes weren't the problem. Maybe arch height is simply an ineffective surrogate for degree of pronation, and alternative methods of shoe assignment should be investigated. One possible method might be to assess foot mobility in terms of the degree of arch collapse rather than just static arch height. A hypermobile foot is one in which the arch collapses considerably upon weight bearing, whereas a hypomobile foot is one in which the arch is very rigid and does not flatten much. You can think of the hypermobile foot as a floppy foot, and the hypomobile foot as a stiff or rigid foot. Conventional wisdom suggests that an arch that collapses excessively will be more likely to overpronate, and thus requires more support in the form of a structured insole or stability/motion control shoe. Conversely, a rigid foot in which the arch collapses only minimally is not good at dissipating shock through pronation, and is thus thought to require greater cushioning.

As our running specialty store sales manager indicated, examination of the degree of arch flattening from sitting to standing is a commonly used method for determining footwear or insole needs—this gives a more direct measure of foot mobility than simply looking at arch height. If the arch flattens too much, you need to prop it up with a supportive insole, right? Sounds reasonable, and the rate at which stores sell inserts is sufficient proof that most runners buy into this logic. However, it would be of interest to know whether looking at arch collapse while standing tells us much of anything about what happens to the arch while one runs, when muscle activity and joint position are considerably different than when one is standing still. Running, after all, is the activity that runners like to participate in—not standing in their socks or bare feet on a pressure mat.

At the University of Virginia SPEED Clinic, Jay Dicharry heads up one of the most high-tech gait analysis labs in the world. In addition to a complex, three-dimensional high-speed camera setup, Dicharry also has at his disposal a custom-built, $750,000 treadmill that can measure in real-time the forces generated as a runner's feet impact the treadmill belt. Dicharry and his small staff spend their days diagnosing the causes of running injuries in their patients and devising plans for how to correct them. He also does footwear validation work for a variety of shoe companies—if you're looking for an expert on the relationship between shoes, biomechanics, anatomy, and injuries, it would be hard to beat the combined package of expertise that Dicharry provides.

Dicharry published a study with colleagues in the *Journal of Orthopaedic & Sports Physical Therapy* in 2009 in which they attempted to examine whether a static (this is when the body is stationary) measure of arch collapse was correlated to actual foot movement while a person is walking or running. According to Dicharry, "The reason for doing this study was that all of the research out there showing when pronation occurs is based on examining rearfoot motion, and the rearfoot is not a comprehensive index of what the entire foot is doing; it's just the rearfoot. We wanted to do a little bit better job" by looking at what the whole foot is doing.

There are a number of methods employed in clinical settings to assess degree of arch collapse. One of these tests is called the functional navicular drop test. Sounds complex, but it's actually quite simple. The navicular is a bone at the top of the arch of the foot, and it can be felt through the skin as a little bump below and in front of the inside of the ankle. Because it is easy to identify, the height of the navicular above the floor can thus be easily measured. In the functional navicular drop test, a clinician measures the height of the navicular while a patient is sitting, and then has the patient bear weight on the foot (by having them stand) and measures the height of the navicular while the arch is compressed. The difference in height is a measure of the degree of arch collapse when the foot bears weight.

Dicharry and his colleagues used the functional navicular drop test (as well as another, slightly more complicated test) to classify individuals as having either hypomobile (minimal arch collapse), neutral (moderate arch collapse), or hypermobile (excessive arch collapse) feet. What they found is that ". . . if you look at static factors you get three very well defined, mutually exclusive categories," says Dicharry. In other words, it's very easy to tell the floppy footed, from the normal footed, from the rigid footed when looking at people who are not moving.

They then filmed these individuals as they walked or ran in the lab so that arch collapse could be determined during dynamic movement. Results showed that despite significant differences in arch collapse between the groups during static testing, arch collapse was identical in all three groups during walking, and the only difference observed during running was a small but significant difference between the hypermobile and hypomobile groups (i.e., the extremes). "When you walk there's really no difference between all of the foot types. They all move about the same," says Dicharry. "If you look at running, only the hypermobile foot types move more . . . it wasn't a big difference." So, only people with floppy feet see increased arch collapse while running, but the difference was actually quite small. In fact, hypermobile individuals on average exhibited only a 1.1 mm greater degree of arch collapse than hypomobile individuals during running. The take-home message from this study was that examining an individual's degree of arch collapse while sitting versus standing still is not a particularly good indicator of what the arch does during actual running; it seems that we can now add degree of arch collapse to the list of questionable diagnostic tools used in the shoe-fitting process.

Given that the idea that flat, floppy feet with collapsing arches require added support is so entrenched in the running world, the results of Dicharry's research might come as a bit of a surprise. How is it that an arch that flattens out considerably when standing can maintain its shape to a much greater degree on the run? Dicharry attributes this to the inherent ability of the body to stabilize joints using muscles. "We're trying to get beyond how much the foot moves, and instead focus on how well you control the foot," says Dicharry. "Let's say I do a navicular drop test on somebody and they've got a lot of motion. Well, if it's somebody with a lot of motion and they've got very good intrinsic foot control, they don't really need a whole lot out of a shoe. If they have good stability, good support, they're gonna be fine." In other words, you can have a flat, floppy foot, but if you can stabilize it well with your foot and leg muscles while you run, you don't need a controlling shoe.

Dicharry goes on: "However, runners with that same foot type, the hypermobile foot type, with poor dynamic control are going to need their shoe to do a lot of things for them. That's kind of what's driven us to get to where we are in footwear. That's definitely something to think about — are the footwear changes that are being done from an industry standpoint actually getting to the root of what needs to be done (which is controlling excessive mobility), or should we all be strengthening their feet? I think everybody should be strengthening their feet." How can this be accomplished? Dicharry thinks that exercises such as practicing standing on one leg, using balance boards, or even skateboarding can more than do the trick. In an interview on the Blue Ridge Outdoors website he goes so far as to say "The stride is all about balance. When you're running, you're always balancing on one leg, so improving that single leg balance is actually the best thing you can do for your running."

Dicharry does believe that shoes can work for those who need them or who don't want to put in the effort and work required to develop internal stability. However, the critical point here is that just because someone has a flat, highly mobile foot does not necessarily mean that he or she needs a motion control shoe. If you combine a foot that is excessively mobile due to loose ligaments or problems with bony articulations with strong muscular support, that person might not need any more shoe than a person with a much less mobile foot. A flat-footed individual who is put in a motion control shoe might be in the entirely wrong shoe when considering that person's ability to internally control stability while running. What's more, wearing a motion control shoe might just interfere with that person's ability to ever develop that internal stability via strengthening of the feet and legs.

Given that examination of arch height and degree of arch collapse may not be effective diagnostic tools for determining pronation, is there any real benefit observing a runner on a treadmill or as he walks or runs across the store's floor? First off, doing an informal exam like this without video is essentially meaningless, as the motions of the feet during running are far too rapid to accurately analyze with the human eye. It's difficult even to assess whether the foot strikes the ground on the heel, midfoot, or forefoot without the assistance of a video camera. Furthermore, even if video is employed, a typical video camera filming at 30 frames/second will only give a limited amount of information—a high-speed camera that films at a minimum of 120 frames/second is best, but few stores have this type of equipment. When Dicharry was asked if he thought that clerks in a shoe store have the ability to effectively determine how much a runner pronates, his response couldn't be more clear: "No, no. Not at all. There's no way that someone can objectively define the pronation state of the foot at all in any shoe store with any of the systems that are out there." This is coming from a biomechanical expert who has a gait lab with 3-D imaging that is far beyond anything you will find in a shoe store.

Dicharry goes on to express frustration with how entrenched the current shoe-fitting process is: "There's sort of the old school hierarchical model of how to match people to shoe types. So the store owner has taught the high school kid who's working there after school how to do the same thing, and they're doing it with you. It's funny—I've literally sent people to stores with a list of shoes. I'll rarely ever send somebody to a store and tell them to buy 'this shoe.' I'll typically tell them, 'Try these five shoes on and see which one you like best.' It cracks me up, you know, I've had folks who've come in for evaluations and they'll say, 'I went to my shoe store and I brought the list that you gave me and the guy wouldn't sell me the shoe. He said I need this.' And I say, 'Well, fine, call the store owner and say thank you for your help, I'm not giving you my business and I'm going to order the shoe on-line.' Shoe store owners need to educate themselves and respond to this. I'm all for supporting the local guy, but they need to educate themselves."

The current pronation-based shoe-fitting paradigm is outdated. Just because it has been standard operating procedure in the past doesn't mean that its use should continue, particularly since there is evidence which suggests that the status quo is ineffective. Individual store owners should be willing to question what they are told by shoe companies, and should investigate the science (or lack thereof) behind the shoe fitting process. Health care professional should do the same, and scientists should put more effort into determining better ways to pair runners up with appropriate shoes, while at the same time doing a better job of educating the public about best practices. It can be hard to change, but with injury rates still at remarkably high levels, perhaps change is what runners need. Indeed, this has already begun to happen, judging by *Runner's World's* Spring 2012 Shoe Guide.

Runner's World Steps into the Future with Its Revised Shoe Guide: Does This Mark the End of the Pronation-Control Paradigm?

For nearly three decades, we organized shoes and reviews into categories: motion control, stability, neutral-cushioned, and performance-training. The format was rooted in the prevailing science, which held that flat-footed runners needed stability features, high-arched runners just needed cushioning, and everyone else fell somewhere in between. But . . . over time that model has grown outdated.

—RUNNER'S WORLD 2012 SPRING SHOE GUIDE

In his opening letter titled "A Big Step Forward," in the March 2012 issue, *Runner's World* Editor-in-Chief David Willey introduced the new direction that the magazine would be taking, indicating that the publication would be moving "away from shoehorning runners into the familiar categories (neutral-cushioned, stability, etc.) that RW codified in the '70s." Willey further writes that "instead of the old categories (so twentieth century!), we are focusing on, well, you. Each quarterly shoe guide will now open with a shoe finder flowchart that quickly takes you to the 'neighborhood' of three to five shoes, depending on your personal needs and likes."

And just what are these "needs and likes" that the new shoe-choice system is based upon? They include the following:

1. Shoe style: traditional vs. minimal.
2. Within the minimal category: some cushioning or very little cushioning.
3. Body Mass Index—above 27 or below 23.
4. Weekly Mileage: less than 18, 18–32, more than 32.
5. Arch Type: low, medium, high.
6. Injury Prone: yes or no.

While the above criteria are a step in the right direction, it's somewhat puzzling to see arch height included in the list, especially since the "Shoe Finder" flowchart in the shoe guide describes the wet-footprint test as a way of determining this, and relates arch type to pronation category. Didn't the above quote indicate that this is a "model that has grown outdated." It's also no certainty that large runners need a special kind of shoe, or that any particular shoe is better for an injury prone runner than any other.

In any case, it's to *Runner's World*'s credit that they were willing to step away from a system that is still widely employed by shoe stores and manufacturers, and one that many runners remain tied to. The magazine should also be praised that it undertook the obviously daunting task of trying to come up with a new method for recommending footwear. There are kinks that still need to be worked out, and there may never be a perfect system for matching shoe to runner, but the new approach represents a seismic shift, especially when a large-circulation publication like *Runner's World* is willing to abandon a system that has been in place for the past thirty or more years. Could this signify the abandonment of the "pronation-control paradigm"? Quite possibly, and the fallout will be incredibly interesting to watch.

Do Shoes Control Pronation?

Let's assume for a moment that a clerk at a shoe store accurately determines that a runner is an overpronator, and fits that runner in a stability shoe. The assumption is that the stability shoe will limit the runner's pronation and thus reduce the risk of injury that overpronation might pose. This begs the question of whether shoes can even effectively control pronation.

In his 2010 book titled *Biomechanics of Sport Shoes*, Benno Nigg provides an extensive review of the literature on the ability of running shoe interventions to control pronation of the foot. He reports that research has shown that shoe interventions can substantially reduce aspects of initial eversion (eversion is an element of pronation that specifically refers to the inward roll of the foot) that occur during the first one-tenth of ground contact, but that these interventions do not substantially reduce total eversion. In a 2001 paper in the *Clinical Journal of Sports Medicine*, Nigg emphasized that results of studies looking at the effects of shoe interventions on running mechanics often yield non-systematic results, meaning that individuals often react differently to a given change in shoe structure. This, combined with the typically small observed effects of such interventions, led him to conclude that "experimental results do not provide any evidence for the claim that shoes, inserts, or orthotics align the skeleton," at least in any consistent manner. Basically, Nigg is suggesting that the ability of shoes to control pronation appears to be small and inconsistent, and that they are not particularly effective at changing the alignment of the skeleton. However, he does acknowledge that "it is known that different shoes do have different total eversion results. Thus, there must be shoe-related characteristics that influence total eversion. These characteristics have not, however, been identified in systematic biomechanical studies." So, some shoe modifications can impact how much the foot rolls inward, we just don't have any good data on which work best. Let's take a look at some of the candidates.

Perhaps the most commonly employed method of attempting to control pronation by running shoe designers is incorporation of a structure known as a medial post into the midsole of a shoe. The midsole is the cushioned portion of the shoe located below your foot that is typically made out of ethylene vinyl acetate (EVA) foam or some type of similar material. The midsole is not to be confused with the outsole, which is the more durable rubber on the bottom of most shoes that directly contacts the ground (the tread). A medial post is a region of the midsole composed of a firmer material on the inner side of the shoe, and a shoe with a medial post is often referred to as having a "dual-density" midsole. If you have a stability or motion control shoe, the medial post can usually be easily identified as a region where the midsole is of a different color, often gray if the rest of the midsole is white. The idea is that you will land on the softer outer margin of the shoe, and as the foot pronates it rolls onto the medial post, which limits further rolling of the foot.

Given his experience evaluating runners in his gait clinic, Jay Dicharry believes that medial posts are not effective tools for controlling pronation:

> *In fact, they can change things for the worse. There are a number of studies out there that show that medial posts actually shift the ground reaction force medially, and increase varus knee torque. {See Chapter 3.} There are a number of publications that show that increasing the varus knee torque increases the risk of medial compartment osteoarthritis. I've not seen a single piece of evidence anywhere that a medial post does anything.*
>
> *Peak deformation/pronation of the foot as defined by the midfoot, looking at the foot in its entirety and not just at the rearfoot, occurs after the heel has left the ground. So if you want to think that your medial post is stopping pronation, it's not even on the ground at the time that you theoretically need it*

Do Feet Pronate Inside Shoes?

In what will likely go down as one of the more gruesome studies of the effects of footwear on running mechanics, Alex Stacoff and colleagues published a paper in a 2000 issue of the *Journal of Biomechanics* that addressed the question of whether measuring pronation through the use of markers on a shoe or on the skin surface (as is typically done) could accurately provide insight regarding the actual movement of the bones inside the foot and leg. This question is of importance as both the shoe and skin can move (or not move) and slide independently of the underlying bones, and measurements of pronation taken from markers placed on these external surfaces might thus be subject to considerable error.

To address this question, Stacoff and colleagues recruited five brave subjects and inserted bone pin markers directly into their calcaneus (heel bone) and tibia (shin bone) under local anesthetic. They then had these subjects run barefoot or in one of several footwear variations {a shoe with three different types of sole—single density foam, dual-density foam, and laterally flared heel—and the dual density shoe with two types of orthotic inserts}. After taking biomechanical measurements during each running trial in each footwear condition, the researchers determined that "differences in the study variables of eversion and tibial rotation between barefoot and shod running were small and not systematic across subjects. The differences between subjects were larger than the differences between shoe and barefoot conditions." This means that variation among individuals was greater than any variation caused by footwear type within a single individual. Thus, they conclude that other studies that have measured aspects of pronation with shoe or skin mounted markers and that have shown differences between barefoot and shod running "did not reflect the movement of the underlying bone."

In practical terms, what this study showed is that although you might observe what appears to be reduced pronation in a motion control shoe, the foot might still pronate inside the shoe just as much as it would inside a neutral shoe or when barefoot. This is in part why gait experts like Dicharry don't believe that it is possible to determine pronation accurately with a simple treadmill and camera setup as commonly employed in a shoe store. It also raises the possibility that what most pronation-control devices in shoes accomplish is limiting movement of the shoe and not of the foot (for example, a medial post might prevent caving in of the midsole as the foot pronates). As with so many aspects of running mechanics, things are not always as simple and straightforward as they seem!

the most. So a medial post is not going to stop motion of the foot—we actually just did a study where we looked at motion of the foot inside the shoe when people are running, and it doesn't stop the foot from moving.

This being said, there are a lot of factors you can change in footwear design that do produce effects. We do validation work for a number of different shoe companies, and I can tell you that when you make changes to the design of footwear, they can have either positive or negative results. Footwear can make a difference; we've got proof to show that. But the medial post is not something we've manipulated to make those changes.

So which aspects of shoe anatomy, so to speak, are actually effective at controlling pronation? Dicharry suggests that some of the most effective variables are the specific location of midsole flex grooves, heel geometry, relative height of the rearfoot vs. forefoot (which determines amount of heel lift), and increased stiffness of the midsole to provide better sensory feedback. He's also quick to point out that shoes can and do work, but that better criteria need to be identified to adequately address the unique needs of each person, and that we need to more deeply investigate which of these aspects of shoe design might work best in a given situation.

Does Pronation Cause Injuries?

It would be quite a shame if you've managed to make it this far through this chapter only to find out that overpronation is not even a significant factor in causing running injuries. After so much time, money and effort spent developing shoes to control this dreaded "wayward" movement of the foot, and with so much angst suffered by runners trying to find the perfect shoe that will prevent their feet from rolling in too much, what if overpronation is really a phantom menace? What if it's not the cursed bogeyman that everyone has been fearing all these years?

Multiple studies have found little if any association between lower extremity alignment or degree of pronation and running injuries, though some have found relationships to specific injury types (it should be noted that study design and method of determining pronation vary widely among studies). In a 1998 review of the scientific literature on the relationship between pronation and running injuries in the journal *Sports Medicine*, Beat Hinterman and Benno Nigg write that the ". . . belief that runners who overpronate have an initially higher risk for sustaining a running-related injury is still widely held by runners and coaches, although there has been no reliable study supporting this." They go on to emphasize that although overpronation might be causally related to running injuries in some instances, they estimate this relationship to be present in "no more than 10% of cases." Once again, Benno Nigg summarizes the current state of knowledge regarding overpronation and running injuries quite well in his 2010 book *Biomechanics of Sports Shoes*:

> . . . the perceived dangers of overpronating and the expectation of resulting injuries resulted in technologies (e.g., dual density midsoles and orthotics) being developed to decrease both the maximum pronation as well as the time to maximum pronation. These products were (wrongly) assumed to be methods for the treatment and prevention of pathologies such as plantar fasciitis, tibial stress fractures, and patella-femoral pain syndrome. Evidence for the effectiveness of such strategies is currently unavailable. It is speculated that there is no such evidence because "overpronation," as it occurs in typical runners, is not a critical predisposition for injuries.
>
> Pronation and supination have long been the "danger variables" hanging over the sport shoe community, but their time as the most important aspects of sport shoe construction is over. Pronation is a natural movement of the foot and "excessive pronation" is a very rare phenomenon. Shoe developers, shoe stores, and medical centres should not be too concerned about "pronation" and "overpronation."

So after this rather long journey through the world of shoe fitting and pronation control, runners everywhere are left to conclude that the methods employed in shoe stores are not very good at determining whether one overpronates, and that the shoes one buys to control overpronation might not be very good at doing so; in fact, for some people these shoes might even be more likely to cause an injury than prevent them. What's more, if Benno Nigg is correct, overpronation might not even be causally associated with the vast majority of running injuries anyway. One is left to wonder why pronation control retains such primacy in the shoe fitting process. Fortunately, driven in part by recent interest in natural running and minimalist footwear, times are slowly changing and footwear innovation is increasing the diversity of options available to individual runners. The days of the pronation-control paradigm, let's hope, are numbered.

Conclusion

After reading this chapter, you might be left asking: "So how do I choose the right shoe?" It's a great question, and one for which there is no easy answer. Matching shoe to runner is complex, and everyone is a bit different. There are guys weighing over 200 pounds who run almost all of their miles barefoot, and fleet-footed folks who have run Boston-qualifying marathons in bulky motion control shoes. Neither should be criticized for their choice; they have found what works for them, and that's all that matters.

The best thing you should do is experiment. Don't be afraid to try what stores or manufacturers might say is "the wrong shoe for you." Consult knowledgeable friends, online sources, and open-minded store clerks who are not tied to broken models. Get to know your personal preferences. Do you like firm cushioning, soft cushioning, or perhaps no cushioning at all? Do you like a flexible sole, or do you prefer a sole that is somewhat stiff? Do you like a shoe that has a heel lift or do you prefer one that is flat? Do you like the narrow fit of a performance racer, or do you prefer a wide toebox that provides freedom of movement for your toes? Do you like a structured upper, or an upper that consists of little more than a layer of fabric to cover your foot? These are all questions to consider, and often the answers can only be determined through experience. Try shoes out—many specialty shops will let you test-drive shoes, and some will let you return a pair that is not working out. If something doesn't feel right, don't ignore it—a shoe should feel comfortable, like it was made just for your foot, and it's better to find another pair than risk doing damage. Searching for the right pair of shoes can take some time, but it can also be a lot of fun. Enjoy the ride!

CHAPTER 7

❧

Foot Strike

Running should be tap, tap, tap . . . not thud, thud, thud.
—Mark Cucuzzella, M.D.

The scene is a smooth dirt road in the Nandi District of Kenya, a hilly, tea-farming region that is the birthplace of long-distance running legends such as Kip Keino, Henry Rono, and Bernard Lagat. A young Kenyan runner, maybe in his early teens, approaches what appears to be a large, chalk outlined rectangle on the road (see Figure 7-1). His posture is erect, upper body oriented vertically, with almost a backward lean at the shoulders. His arms are bent at the elbow about 90 degrees, hands held in a relaxed, lightly clenched fist. The runner's right leg stretches forward, knee almost fully extended as he reaches for the ground. His bare foot, still floating several inches above the dirt surface, is slightly plantar-flexed (foot angled down relative to the shin), positioning his sole parallel to the ground. The curvature of the lateral arch of his foot is distinct, a sloping concavity between his protruding heel and the ball behind his little toe. His toes extend upward, reaching toward the sky as he comes in for a landing.

As the young boy floats in toward the surface, his hip begins to extend just a bit, rotating his thigh slightly down and back, and his knee begins to flex. In contrast, his ankle seems to hold its position. Flexing of the knee causes his shin to assume a more vertical position relative to the ground. As a result, the sole of his foot, initially parallel to the ground surface, is now inclined downward from heel to ball. Initial touchdown is thus made on the forefoot, just behind the little toe. Contact by the toes follows shortly thereafter, and then his heel comes down, stretching the calf muscles and Achilles tendon like rubber bands. As the boy's body begins to travel over his now planted foot, his knee continues to flex, but its movement is now joined by rotation about the ankle. His ankle dorsiflexes (foot angled up relative to the shin), further stretching the calf and Achilles tendon as the angle between foot and shin becomes more acute, and his hip extends, pulling the thigh backward as the weight of his body passes over.

As his left leg swings forward, the stance leg continues to extend at the hip, but his knee now starts to extend as well, and his foot begins to plantarflex at the ankle—the leg is straightening out in preparation to propel the runner into the next step. As his right leg continues to extend out behind him, the boy's heel comes up off of the ground, leaving the forefoot and toes in sole contact with the surface below. His thigh is now extended slightly behind a line drawn from shoulder to hip, and his knee is almost locked in a fully extended position. Finally, his toes lift off the ground, and the runner is fully airborne, the left leg preparing to go through the same series of maneuvers.

What we've described here is the fluid, natural running form of someone who has never before worn shoes, as captured on slow-motion video by Dr. Daniel Lieberman.

Several years later and over 7,000 miles away in the small city of Concord, New Hampshire, a middle-aged male runner is competing in a five-kilometer race (see Figure 7-2). He makes the final turn onto the asphalt road leading to the finish line, which is just a few blocks away. His form is unremarkable when compared to the other runners passing by, but in certain distinctive ways it contrasts starkly with that of the Kenyan boy described above. He's wearing bulky running shoes with a sole composed of several centimeters of foam cushioning, with additional padding underneath the heel. As with the Kenyan boy, he initially approaches the ground with an extended knee, but below the ankle something is

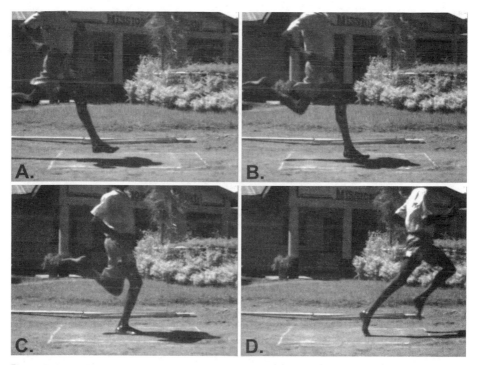

Figure 7-1. Running form of a habitually barefoot Kenyan adolescent on a dirt road. Reproduced with permission from video taken by Dr. Daniel Lieberman.

dramatically different. Rather than being plantarflexed, his foot forms an angle of about 90 degrees with his extended lower leg, and the sole of his shoe from heel to toe is inclined almost 45 degrees relative to the ground. As his foot approaches the ground, another difference becomes apparent—his ankle holds position, just as it did in the barefoot Kenyan, but his knee remains almost completely locked as well. As a result, he contacts the ground firmly on the very back, outer portion of the heel, with his lower leg still extended far out in front of his knee. His foot remains inclined approximately 45 degrees relative to the asphalt surface when he touches down. The cushioning below the heel compresses rapidly upon contact, and the heel is forced upward. The resulting rotation about the ankle causes the forefoot to slap down quickly. Once the foot is planted, the motions are once again similar to those of the young Kenyan as he propels himself into his next stride.

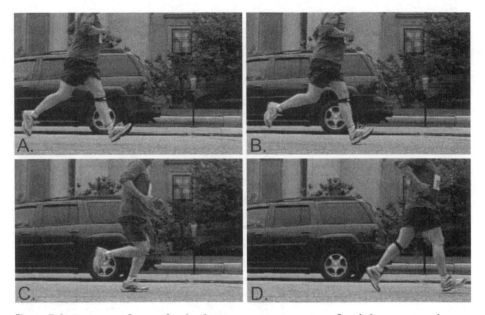

Figure 7-2. Running form of a shod American runner in a five-kilometer road race.

As we have discussed in previous chapters, the mode of interaction between the human foot and the ground has changed considerably over time. The average person went from being habitually barefoot, just like the Kenyan boy described above, to wearing fairly simple shoes or sandals, to in the past several hundred years going about in shoes that have little if any respect for the anatomy of the human foot. Running shoes have followed a somewhat similar evolution—from simple leather shoes with little protection under the sole, to high-tech devices made of mostly synthetic materials, typically with a thick wedge of foam between the foot and the ground. In this chapter we will examine more closely the effect that these changes in footwear design have had on the way that we run.

Let's start with a simple experiment. First, take off your shoes and go stand at the top of a flight of stairs. Now, walk slowly down the stairs and when you get to the last step, hop on to the floor. Now jog in place for ten seconds. Easy, right?

Now, do this series of activities again, making careful note of which part of your foot contacts the ground first with each step. We're willing to bet that on every single step you took, initial contact was made on the forefoot, just behind the toes. Now try it a third time and try to consciously make first contact on your heel (be careful not to tumble down the stairs!). Pretty tough, huh?

Why is it that without even consciously thinking about it, your body chose to land on the forefoot during each of the above activities? The answer is quite simple—walking down steps, jumping, and running in place are all activities that involve the feet supporting your entire body weight as it impacts the ground, and the bony heel is a pretty lousy shock absorber.

When your body really needs to absorb shock, you land on your forefoot, and you naturally use the stretch of your calf muscles and Achilles tendon to gently lower you to the ground. What's more, as these muscles and tendons stretch, they store energy like a rubber band, which can be released to propel you into your next step forward. It should be noted that none of the above activities is a perfect mimic of the dynamic motion that occurs when you walk or run, where forward momentum and our ability to roll over our feet at the ankle joint allows for more variation in footfall pattern (for example, the typical heel-toe human walking gait), but the point stands: when a soft landing is needed, you generally don't want to impact on your heels.

How does this simple experiment relate to running? Running is a repetitive impact sport, many people get injured doing it, and one of the most highly variable aspects of the human running gait is the foot strike—specifically, which part of the foot makes initial contact with the ground while one runs. Observations like those made when jumping up and down or running in place would suggest that landing on the forefoot might be the best way to dissipate impact force during running.

Recent studies have shown that adoption of a forefoot landing is in fact what habitual barefoot runners tend to do when they run. However, shoe design has long focused on protecting the heel by adding an elevated wedge of cushion underneath it, and most shod runners do in fact tend to land on their heels. The implications of this difference between typical barefoot and shod foot strike patterns have been the source of much recent discussion and argument in the running community. Indeed, debate regarding how the foot should optimally strike the ground to maximize performance or reduce injury risk has simmered among coaches, scientists, and runners alike for decades, and to this day there remains little consensus. Though some individuals hold strong opinions on this topic, it's quite possible that there may in fact be no single answer that applies to all situations and for all runners.

Our approach here is not so much to provide any definitive one-size-fits-all answer, but rather to examine and try to make some sense of what we currently know about how the foot strikes the ground while running, why it might be important, and how it might be altered by the shoes that one wears.

The Variable Running Foot Strike

The running foot strike is just one small part of the overall running gait, so let's begin by clearly defining each of the three possible categories into which a given running foot strike might be placed:

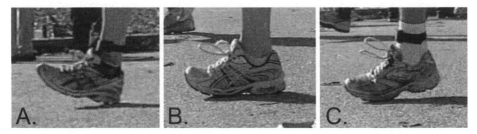

Figure 7-3. Representative images of the three major foot strike categories taken from high speed video recorded at mile 6 of the 2009 Manchester (NH) City Marathon. **A.** Heel strike. **B.** Midfoot strike. **C.** Forefoot strike.

1. Rearfoot—initial contact between the foot and the ground is made somewhere on the outer portion of the heel of the foot/shoe (see Figure 7-3A).
2. Midfoot—the heel and the forefoot contact simultaneously along the outer margin of the foot/shoe. This category is sometimes referred to as full-foot or flat-foot strike (see Figure 7-3B).
3. Forefoot—initial contact is made on the outer side of the front half of the foot/shoe, usually along the pad behind the little toe. The heel typically comes down shortly thereafter (see Figure 7-3C).

It's important to recognize that considerable variation exists within these categories, and that foot strike classification is perhaps better viewed as a spectrum rather than a series of mutually exclusive groupings. For example, a heel strike can occur roughly anywhere along the rear one-third of the foot/shoe, and foot position at contact can vary from one in which the sole of the shoe is oriented at almost a 45-degree angle to the ground, to one where the foot is nearly flat at contact, with the heel touching down only slightly before the forefoot. A forefoot strike typically occurs as previously described—initial contact at the outer forefoot, followed quickly thereafter by the heel touching down (commonly referred to as a ball-heel-ball gait). Some runners, however, land up near the toes and never allow the heel to touch the ground. Even a midfoot strike can vary in the amount of supination/inversion (inward bending) of the foot at ground contact. What's more, each foot strike type can be accompanied by varying orientations of joints higher up in the leg. For example, some people land with an almost fully extended knee, like our 5K runner, whereas others tend to have considerably more bend in their joints, like the barefoot Kenyan boy. All of these factors need to be kept in mind during any discussion of the running foot strike.

A Brief History of Foot-Strike Recommendations

Looking back through history, one can find any number of contrasting viewpoints on which foot strike type (heel, midfoot, or forefoot) should be adopted by runners. For example, in his classic, bestselling 1977 book *The Complete Book of Running*, Jim Fixx writes:

> *Each foot should strike the ground at the heel and roll forward, finally pushing off with the toes. If this feels unnatural, try landing flatfooted. Don't run on your toes; you'll only get sore calf muscles and possibly strain your Achilles tendons.*

In the *Serious Runner's Handbook*, published in 1978, elite ultrarunner Tom Osler says the following:

> *When the foot first makes contact with the ground, it should be with the heel, and not the ball of the foot. The best way to determine how you land is to examine the soles of your shoes. If the heel area is wearing most rapidly, then you are landing properly. If the area near the ball of the foot is wearing out first (especially behind the little toe), then you*

are landing too far forward. By landing on the ball of the foot, the shock of ground contact is absorbed in the calf muscles. This is tiring in very long runs, but tolerable in sprints and middle-distance races under one mile. By landing on the heel, the calf is rested and the shock is absorbed in the bones.

In his book *Chi Running*, author Danny Dreyer advocates a midfoot strike, arguing that while using his method:

. . . you are no longer "braking" because your feet are landing in a midfoot strike and moving toward the rear when they strike the ground. This allows your legs to swing out behind you as soon as your feet touch the ground, radically reducing the amount of impact to your knees and quads . . . The midfoot strike is exactly how it sounds. You're not landing on only the heel or the ball of the foot. Your whole foot lands, with the pressure equally balanced from front to back and side to side.

Current American half-marathon record holder Ryan Hall is also an advocate of midfoot striking. In an on-line technique instruction video produced through his Steps Foundation, Hall states the following:

Basically what I'm looking for in all my drills and running is keeping this foot dorsiflexed as I cycle it through the run, and then as the foot strikes, hitting flat footed so that it's like a spring—it's already coiled up, and it's already ready to explode off the ground. It also keeps your energy so that it's going into the ground and propelling you forward and not right back at you like if you were to land really high on your heels like you see a lot of people doing. A lot of energy is coming right back at you in the other direction—it's actually a lot harder to run that way.

Joe Henderson, author of multiple books on running, and former editor and long-time columnist at *Runner's World*, provides the following description of ideal running footplant in his book *Running 101*:

Landing on midfoot, not heel-first; dropping quickly to heel and up again for toe-off, not stiff-ankled; knee slightly flexed, not locked. {Authors' note: this is a description of a forefoot strike using the commonly applied definitions.}

Gordon Pirie, an exceptional British distance runner from the 1950's (he set five world records during his career and was a silver medalist in the 10,000 meters at the 1956 Melbourne Olympics), believes that a runner should employ a forefoot striking gait. In his book *Running Fast and Injury Free*, Pirie writes:

> *The nerves conveying tactile sensation from the foot are predominantly located in the forefoot. When the ball of the foot touches the ground, these nerves "alert" the muscles of the legs, which involuntarily react to absorb the shock of landing. If a person hits the ground heel-first, this reaction of the leg muscles will be considerably less, and consequently more shock will be experienced at the point of contact of the foot, and be transmitted to the bones of the leg. This jarring is guaranteed eventually to cause injury to the ankle, knee and/or hip joints.*
>
> *It is therefore important that a runner lands on the forward portion of the foot, with the knee slightly bent, and with the foot placed beneath the body. By doing so, the runner will make use of the body's own efficient shock absorbers—the arch of the foot, the calf muscles, and the quadriceps muscles in the thighs—and in this way reduce the stress experienced by the heel, shin bone, knee joint, thigh bone and hip joint. It is these areas which are stressed the most when the heel strikes the ground.*

Perhaps the most diplomatic approach was expressed by legendary University of Oregon track coach Bill Bowerman and his coauthor W. E. Harris, in their popular 1967 book *Jogging*:

> *There are three basic methods of foot strike, but no one method that you must use. Study each and choose the one that is most comfortable, efficient and works best for you.*

They go on to describe the differences between heel-to-toe, flat-foot, and ball-of-the-foot striking. They indicate that heel-toe is the "least tiring over long distances and the least wearing on the rest of the body," whereas "the ball-of-the-foot technique sometimes produces soreness since the muscles must remain in contraction for a longer period of time than heel-to-toe or flat-foot."

In a 1971 *Sports Illustrated* article titled "The Secrets of Speed," Bowerman further elaborates on his thoughts about foot strike:

There are two basic ways in which the foot may strike the ground. The most common, as well as the most comfortable and efficient, is for the foot to hit flat, or possibly back toward the heel, and then roll forward across the ball. The second, which is used primarily by a runner needing a short, explosive burst of speed, is to land on the ball of the foot and stay up on it throughout the entire stride. There are runners who are endowed with sufficiently limber ankles to be able to hit on the ball of the foot and then settle back on the heel, but this is extremely rare.

Bowerman further warns that ". . . {for} those who run up on the ball of the foot: this practice puts pressure on the arch of the foot as well as on the bones and muscles. If performed for distances over a few hundred yards, the chances are it will cause knotting and fatigue in the calf muscles, and there is the possibility of various injuries."

Given the wide variety found among the recommendations provided by these running experts, it's easy to forgive the average runner who gets confused when trying to figure out just what his or her feet should be doing!

How Do Most Runners Strike the Ground with Their Feet?

Given the welter of contradiction and disagreement about which foot strike pattern is most appropriate for runners, another approach is to simply observe runners and figure out what most of them do. Over the years, several studies have done just that, and the results have generally pointed overwhelmingly in one direction.

Two of the most comprehensive studies of foot strike patterns in distance runners were conducted over two decades apart (it should be noted that running shoe design went through many changes between these studies). First, a study published by B. A. Kerr and colleagues in a sports shoe conference proceedings from 1983 looked at foot strike patterns in runners in a ten-kilometer road race in Calgary, as well as at two points in a marathon (at twenty kilometers and thirty-five kilometers) in Edmonton. It found that on average at the three filming locations, about 80 percent of runners made first contact on their heel, while almost all remaining runners landed on their midfoot. The study observed that frequency of midfoot striking increased among the faster runners in its sample (nearly evenly split between heel vs. midfoot in the fastest sample). Perhaps most interestingly, the data showed only two forefoot strikers out of the more than 700 runners who were filmed, and both were among the faster runners in the final stages of the 10K.

A second study was conducted in Japan by Hiroshi Hasegawa of Ryukoku University and colleagues. The authors of this 2007 study in the *Journal of Strength and Conditioning Research* set out to determine foot strike patterns (as well as other gait parameters) during the 2004 Sapporo International Half-Marathon. This was a highly competitive race, with elite caliber runners, and Hasegawa filmed them in slow motion as they passed at the fifteen kilometer mark.

Foot Strike in Contemporary Recreational Runners

To determine how average, everyday runners typically contact the ground in a race, I decided to task a group of my undergraduate research students at Saint Anselm College with filming the Manchester (New Hampshire) City Marathon in November, 2009. We filmed the race at roughly the six and twenty mile markers using a high-speed video camera that could record at 300 frames per second. Based on the video footage obtained from the six mile mark, we determined left and right foot strike patterns of 936 marathon, half-marathon, and relay runners, most of whom would be considered of recreational or sub-elite ability (for reference, the average finish time for the sample of full-marathon runners that we analyzed was 3:57:31). Of these, 88.9 percent were classified as rearfoot strikers, 3.4 percent were midfoot strikers, 1.8 percent were forefoot strikers, and 5.9 percent of runners exhibited discrete foot strike asymmetry (meaning a different foot strike pattern on each foot). Although an accurate quantitative analysis of foot strike angles was not possible, subjective analysis suggested that about 50 percent of heel strikes could be considered "extreme."

Because we obtained additional footage from the twenty mile mark, we were able to compare foot strike patterns of 286 individual marathon runners between the two race locations. We observed increased frequency of rearfoot striking at twenty miles as compared to the six mile location—in other words, a large percentage of runners switched from midfoot and forefoot foot strikes at six miles to rearfoot strikes at twenty miles, presumably due to muscular fatigue. The results of this study were published in a late 2011 issue of the *Journal of Sports Sciences*.   —PML

Overall, 74.9 percent of the 283 (248 men, 35 women) runners that Hasegawa filmed were classified as rearfoot strikers (80 percent of women, 74.2 percent of men), 23.7 percent were midfoot strikers (17.1 percent of women, 25.6. percent of men), and only 1.4 percent were forefoot strikers (2.9 percent of women, 0.2 percent of men). The researchers went on to classify runners into fifty-person subgroups by finishing times to look at whether foot strike patterns varied with speed. They found that the frequency of runners adopting a midfoot or forefoot strike was relatively higher in both men and women in the faster subgroups. However, in almost all subgroups rearfoot striking remained most common—for example, in the fastest group of fifty men (averaging a 15:17 per 5K pace), 62 percent were heel strikers, 36 percent were midfoot strikers, and only 2 percent were forefoot strikers. So, even in elite-level half marathoners, rearfoot striking is the most commonly observed pattern.

One difficulty with all of these foot strike studies is that they were conducted well after the advent of the modern, cushioned running shoe. Even racing flats similar to those likely worn by the racers in Japan typically have cushioning and a moderately lifted heel (ironically, "flats" are rarely flat). Thus, it's difficult to know whether it was the introduction of shoes themselves, or the addition of cushioning or a lifted heel to the running shoe that might have led runners away from typical barefoot running form exhibited by the Kenyan runner on the dirt road. And while videos of runners prior to 1970 are available, most were filmed at too slow of a speed to accurately analyze the rapid motions that occur during the running stride. However, there is one study that offers a tantalizing glimpse of how runners' feet typically contacted the ground prior to 1970.

In 1964, a fascinating study by German national track coach Toni Nett was published in the technical track and field journal *Track Technique*. The paper was actually a translated English synthesis of an article that had appeared previously in a 1952 issue of the German publication *Die Lehre der Leichtathletik*. Nett analyzed foot strike patterns of elite runners from the 1950's (included in his sample was the great Czech runner Emil Zatopek, who won gold medals in the 5,000 meters, 10,000 meters and marathon at the 1952 Helsinki Olympics). Nett was able to film these runners in high-level competitions at 64 frames/second—not particularly high-speed video by modern standards, but fast enough to get an idea of what the runners' feet were doing. His reason for doing this was to "throw light on the problem of more than fifty years standing: how the foot is planted." This statement implies that debate about foot strike stretched back to the early 1900s! Nett indicated that there had long been a polarized debate among coaches, with some insisting that "all runners at all distances plant the foot heel first," while others insisted that "the foot is planted exclusively on the ball by all runners at all distances." Nett was interested in determining which of these viewpoints was correct, or whether perhaps foot strike varied by speed or distance run.

Based on his analysis of runners in events ranging from 100 meters to the marathon, Nett recognized the following:

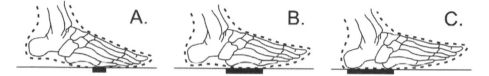

Figure 7-4. Foot strike diagrams adapted from Toni Nett's 1964 article in *Track Technique*. **A.** Active or dynamic ball plant. **B.** Metatarsal plant. **C.** Passive or static heel-metatarsus plant. Thick black bars indicate location of initial contact between the foot and ground.

1. All runners, regardless of event or specific foot strike type, initially planted the foot somewhere on the outside edge; in other words, they landed on an initially supinated/inverted foot.
2. The 100-meter and 200-meter runners initially contacted high on the outside edge of the ball of the foot, including the joints of the little toe (see Figure 7-4A). The 400-meter runners contacted the ground slightly further back along the outer edge of the ball of the foot from the sprinters. Nett called this the "active or dynamic ball plant."
3. The 800-meter runners typically landed along the length of the fifth metatarsal, with the heels and toes slightly off the ground at contact (see Figure 7-4B). Nett called this the "metatarsal plant."
4. 1500-meter runners landed in a manner similar to either the 800 meter runners or in a manner similar to marathon runners—in other words, this is a distance where runners exhibited some variability in foot strike type (see Figures 7-4B and 7-4C).

5. The runners in events ranging from longer than 1,500 meters to the marathon contacted "with the outside edge of the arch between the heel and metatarsus (see diagram "C")." Emil Zatopek was included in this group. Nett called this the "passive or static heel-metatarsus plant." He found only one exception to this—one runner landed on the ball.

So how do Nett's categories translate into modern foot strike terminology? Based on Nett's illustrations (Figure 7-4), it appears that the sprinter's foot strike (Figure 7-4A) is what is commonly referred to as toe running, or an extreme forefoot strike. The 800-meter to 1,500-meter foot strike (Figure 7-4B) is what's typically referred to as a forefoot strike since the heel does not make contact upon initial foot plant. The 1,500-meters to marathon foot strike (Figure 7-4C) corresponds to a midfoot strike since both the heel and base of the fifth metatarsal make contact simultaneously. This category might also include mild heel strikes, but it's hard to be absolutely certain from Nett's descriptions. (The base of the fifth metatarsal is located about midway from the heel to the base of the little toes, and if you try to place your foot down so that it contacts at both the heel and this location simultaneously, you will see that contact is roughly along the entire outer margin of the foot.)

Based upon his observations, Nett made the following conclusions:

1. The sprinting foot strike allows for a fast pace, but is "rather energy-consuming."
2. The "metatarsal plant" is intermediate in terms of strength requirement and is thus suitable for middle distances.
3. The "static heel-metatarsus plant" is an endurance gait since it requires the least energy per step, but it is not suitable for high speed.

Nett emphasized that foot-plant is correlated strongly with pace, and he recounted his observation that when sprinters run in a more long-distance situation, they adopt a foot plant like that seen in marathoners. Because of this, he cautioned readers not to make their own conclusions on the foot plant of individuals solely based on still race photos since a middle distance runner sprinting to the finish line will adopt a sprinter's foot strike (you need high-speed video to truly provide an accurate assessment of foot strike). Similarly, a fatigued recreational marathoner crossing the finish line may not be exhibiting the same form as he or she had earlier in the race (so don't let your embarrassing form in finish-line photos get you down; you're not always *that* runner!).

Nett further wrote "foot-plant evidently follows laws that lie outside the person, that lie in the rate of running speed." The foot strikes that he observed were so consistent in the different events that the speed at which an individual was running was the most accurate predictor of how the foot first contacted the ground. In contrast, other aspects of running form (trunk, arms, head) were so variable that "not even remotely can so uniform a picture be obtained." He considered these other factors to be elements of individual style rather than related to speed or distance.

What conclusions can be drawn from these studies of foot strike patterns in runners? First, most shod distance runners filmed after 1980 were heel-strikers, and frequency of heel striking appears to be greater among slower runners. Second, forefoot striking was rare among shod long-distance runners (even among elite marathoners in the 1950s), and fatigued forefoot strikers often reverted to a heel-striking gait late in a long-distance race like a marathon (so forefoot striking might not be an ideal gait for the average marathon racer). Third, based upon Nett's analysis, elite runners in the 1950's appeared not to have exhibited an extreme heel strike like that frequently observed in the typical recreational runner in modern shoes. What's more, if Nett's "passive or static heel-metatarsus plant" is in fact equivalent to a midfoot strike (using modern terminology), then pure heel striking of any kind may have been rare among elites in the 1950's (though one might suspect that category probably included midfoot strikers and mild heel strikers).

Given the patterns that have been observed, it might be tempting to generalize, as Nett suggested, that foot strike type is primarily a function of how fast the runner is moving. Speed obviously plays a big role, as anyone who watches a 100-meter race can easily observe that a sprinter exhibits a very different foot strike type than a marathoner. However, would 100-meter world record holder Usain Bolt revert to a heavy heel strike while on a leisurely cool-down jog? Unlikely, and post-race videos of Bolt indicate that he continues to midfoot or forefoot strike on his cool-down lap. Though foot strike may change to some degree, and heel striking might occur, elites don't suddenly start mashing the ground when they are jogging slowly. Similarly, some mid-pack marathon runners do in fact forefoot strike, and scientific studies have shown that when speed is held constant, location of initial foot strike among individuals can occur anywhere along the rear 60 percent of the outer margin of the shoe. Thus, speed clearly cannot solely explain the full range of foot strike types observed among runners.

What other factors might be important in determining foot strike type? Running surface is likely one, as factors such as hardness and irregularity will require some adaptation of foot orientation relative to the ground underfoot. There's also a runner's flexibility, neuromuscular control, and training background. And then there's the most potentially critical factor, and perhaps one of the easiest to modify: the runner's footwear (or lack thereof).

It's Gotta' Be the Shoes!

It seems reasonable to think that for a given combination of surface and speed, humans should exhibit a fairly stereotypical running style—we all do belong to the same species after all. However, humans have introduced a major complicating factor that can have a profound effect on how we run under any given set of conditions—we have created shoes. By wearing shoes, a runner introduces an artificial filter (the sole) between his or her feet and the ground. Since shoes come in seemingly innumerable varieties, each might change the foot-ground interface in its own subtle way. What's more, each individual has a personal physical activity background and shoe-wearing history that have likely left their mark in some way on the anatomy of the legs and feet. As such, it is likely impossible to identify a stereotypical or default human running form among a group of shod runners, even if they are running at the same speed, on the same ground surface, and are otherwise physically fit, active, and healthy.

Perhaps the closest glimpse we have of what we might call "natural" human running form is provided by physically fit, active individuals who have never worn shoes and who are running on a natural surface, much like the barefoot Kenyan boy on the dirt road whose form was described at the opening of this chapter. Footwear represents a relatively modern change to an evolutionary and developmental norm (we aren't born with shoes on our feet), and it's only relatively recently that scientists have begun to address the question of how shoes influence running form.

Daniel Lieberman's research from the rift valley of Kenya found that habitually unshod individuals and those who started wearing shoes only later in life almost always landed on their midfoot or forefoot while running. Conversely, Lieberman found that American adults who run all of their miles in typical cushioned training shoes landed on their heel 100 percent of the time. Both groups were performing the same activity—running—but the biomechanical result was very different.

What explains this difference? Was it simply the addition of shoes, or might running speed, age, surface, or some other factor have been involved? After all, that same group of habitually shod, heel-striking American runners continued to do so 83 percent of the time when they took their shoes off. A similar pattern was observed for the group of habitually shod Kenyan adolescents that Lieberman examined—they tended to heel strike regardless of what they did or did not have on their feet.

Some insight regarding the role of footwear in influencing foot strike type can be gained by looking at individuals who grew up shod, but made a decision later in life to go barefoot. The back-to-barefoot American adults that Lieberman examined landed on their forefoot 75 percent of the time when barefoot; but when shod, they exhibited a 50-50 split between heel striking and midfoot/forefoot striking. The results for the back-to-barefooters suggest that perhaps there is a learning component involved when it comes to running form, and that adaptations to footwear, or lack thereof, may take a bit of time to set in.

The Importance of Acclimation

One significant limitation of many of the existing biomechanical studies of running form is that they often fail to account for the possibility that form change in response to a footwear intervention is a prolonged process that requires a certain amount of time for acclimation or learning to occur. For example, a researcher might take a habitually shod runner, ask him to remove his shoes, and have him run on a treadmill or down a runway without much of an acclimation period to being barefoot. Without sufficient time for adaptation and learning, it seems unlikely that a researcher will observe a fluid representation of barefoot running form in the test subject. This is particularly problematic in studies of running efficiency, as individuals will likely be less efficient if asked to perform a novel movement pattern on the spot. As an analogy, think about how hard it is to throw a ball with your non-dominant hand, or to type for the first time on a keyboard of non-standard size (recall the first time you attempted to type out a text message on a cell phone!). You will surely improve with practice, but initial attempts will likely be awkward and ineffective. Similarly, running barefoot is an entirely different sensory experience than running in shoes, and it would not be surprising if initial attempts felt a bit strange. It would also not be surprising if you initially adopted the form that your body knows and that has become ingrained in its muscle memory—for most, that form is one that has been fine tuned by many years of running in cushioned shoes.

In an interview with Amby Burfoot on the *Runner's World Peak Performance* blog, Jay Dicharry shared his thoughts about the importance of past experience and muscle memory. "You move the way you do because it feels normal," says Dicharry, "but what if the way you learned to move wasn't the best?" He uses the example of a runner who has a persistent calf injury: "Maybe you had some nagging soreness in your calf and you altered your stride a bit. This change then became permanent and now you've got chronic something-or-other that you just can't get rid of." In other words, compensating for a chronic injury teaches you to run in a different way, and this new way of running becomes your new normal. The only problem is that the new normal creates an issue somewhere else. "Practice makes perfect," says Dicharry, only you want to make sure that the running form that you practice is not one that is going to get you hurt.

Let's consider for a moment the role of acclimation in gait retraining. Suppose you're a traditionally shod runner who wishes to work on modifying or refining your form by incorporating a bit of barefoot running into your weekly routine. On your first barefoot run, you'll likely initially adopt your typical shod running form—it's what you know, and it's what your body finds most comfortable. For most people this form would include a fairly prominent heel strike. However, if you are running on a hard surface like an asphalt road, your body will very quickly adapt because smashing your bare heel into a hard surface is not a sustainable way to run (far from it!). So, perhaps you'll first move to a milder heel strike as your body searches for a better way to deal with the impact stimulus—a mild heel strike is similar to what you're used to, but dampens the impact down a bit. As the stimulus is repeated, your feet might start to adopt a midfoot or forefoot strike, allowing the calf muscles to act as natural springs to cushion your landing just as they do when you hop in place. You're now running in a new way, and it's probably a way of running that you haven't utilized since you were a kid running barefoot in the backyard. It probably feels strange and awkward, but it works—you're running on a very hard surface, and it no longer hurts.

The catch with this approach to gait modification is that changing a long-practiced and complex movement pattern like your running form can be difficult, as it requires alteration of what psychologists refer to as procedural memory—this is the type of memory that allows you to learn how to perform actions and complex motor skills (the phrase "muscle memory" is sometimes used here). Every one of us learns how to run at a very young age, and we generally don't need any instruction in how to do so. However, most individuals in the developed world probably learned this skill with some type of shoes on their feet, and thus the specific nature of their running form is likely influenced to some degree by their childhood footwear.

How you ran in childhood might play a big role in how you now run as an adult. For example, former marathon world record holder Haile Gebreselassie has a distinct arm carry on one side that he attributes to having carried his books with that arm while he ran to school as a kid in Ethiopia. Clearly Geb isn't carrying books when he runs these days, but his childhood routine left its indelible imprint on his adult running form.

Research does exist which shows that footwear can alter stride characteristics even in children. A systematic review of the effects of footwear on the walking and running gaits of children published in 2011 in the *Journal of Foot and Ankle Research* concluded with the following statement: "With shoes, children walk faster by taking longer steps with greater ankle and knee motion and increased tibialis anterior activity. Shoes reduce foot motion and increase the support phases of the gait cycle. During running, shoes reduce swing phase leg speed, attenuate some shock and encourage a rearfoot strike pattern. The long-term effect of these changes on growth and development are currently unknown." If shoes influence the mechanics of walking and running in children, could this lead to the development of an ingrained muscle memory that is very difficult to change in adulthood? Perhaps. Some runners will forefoot strike no matter what shoes they wear; and others will continue to heel strike even when barefoot (even a few of the habitually unshod Kenyan children that Lieberman filmed were heel strikers). However, others seem to be more adaptable and are capable of making a faster transition. Nonetheless, though physical limitations may play a role in determining what the feet can do, it's intriguing to consider the fact that psychology could be involved as well. What we (or our parents) put on our feet in childhood might play a big role in the development of our individual running form, and movement patterns that we develop early in childhood might be quite difficult for us to "un-learn" as adults.

Much of this discussion so far regarding running form acclimation to changes in footwear has been based upon a mixture of speculation and informed observation. However, there are some hints in the scientific literature on running mechanics that strongly suggest that motor learning may play an important role when it comes to adapting to changes in what you do or do not put on your feet. Once again, we turn our attention to the research of Dr. Daniel Lieberman.

One of the often-overlooked aspects of Lieberman's 2010 barefoot running study in the journal *Nature* was the supplementary data. Within this addendum was a section about a study he conducted looking specifically at the question of "if and/or how habitually shod RFS (rear-foot strike) runners change their strike when they transition from wearing running shoes to minimal footwear." Lieberman and his colleagues recruited fourteen runners and provided each of them with a pair of Vibram FiveFingers Sprint shoes (the study was partially funded by Vibram). The FiveFingers are basically nothing more than a minimally cushioned "foot glove," with individual pockets for each toe. The subjects were provided instruction to increase distance in the shoes very gradually over the course of six weeks, to a maximum of sixteen to twenty kilometers per week. They were provided no instruction on how to run in the FiveFingers, so any change that occurred was due to experience running in the shoes, and thus could be attributed to acclimation/learning. Subjects were each filmed prior to the six-week trial period, and then again after the six weeks were over.

The results of the study showed that form changed significantly over the course of the six weeks of running in the Vibram FiveFingers Sprints. Foot strike patterns changed as follows:

Strike Type	Week 0 % subjects (# subjects)	Week 6 % subjects (# subjects)
Rearfoot	72 (10)	36 (5)
Midfoot	14 (2)	0
Forefoot	14 (2)	57 (8)
Toe Strike (no heel contact at all)	0	7 (1)

If we assume that the two forefoot strikers at the outset remained forefoot strikers after six weeks, then seven of the twelve individuals changed their foot strike from either rearfoot or midfoot to forefoot/toe after transitioning to the barefoot-style shoes. Five individuals remained heel strikers, but results showed that the runners on average struck the ground with a more plantarflexed foot (flatter foot plant), so their heel strike may have been less pronounced. These results indicate that over the course of six weeks, some of these runners "learned" how to run in these shoes in a way that differed from their initial pattern.

Lieberman's findings are supported by a 2009 study in the *Journal of Sports Medicine & Physical Fitness*, which compared the biomechanics of experienced barefoot runners while running barefoot, in Vibrams, and in traditional cushioned shoes. Study authors Roberto Squadrone and Claudio Gallozzi from the Institute of Sport Medicine and Sport Science of the Italian Olympic National Committee found that when running in Vibram FiveFingers, the runners had a significantly more plantarflexed foot at ground contact when compared to running in standard cushioned shoes. Thus, the adaptations observed by Lieberman are perfectly in line with what experienced barefoot/minimalist runners do. Furthermore, a more recent 2011 study sponsored by the American Council on Exercise (ACE) found that 50 percent of sixteen women who ran in the Vibram FiveFingers for two weeks adopted a forefoot strike landing pattern (all sixteen were heel strikers in typical running shoes).

Despite these small sample sizes, what all of these studies suggest is that there is an adaptive response to running in an ultra-minimal shoe like the Vibram FiveFingers, and that this response may take time to manifest itself. The fact that some people alter foot strike pattern after several weeks of running in Vibrams, whereas others do not, could reflect the fact that some individuals will heel strike no matter what. Alternatively, it could be evidence that adaptation occurs at different rates in different people—this would not be surprising, because when it comes to biology, variation is usually the norm. It would be interesting to know if those who remained heel strikers in these studies would eventually adopt a different foot strike if allowed more time to practice running in the barefoot-style shoes. There's clearly a need for longer-term adaptation studies.

The results of these acclimation studies also indicate that skepticism is warranted when comparing running form in individuals based upon an "on the spot" change in footwear condition. Furthermore, they show that if you have the goal of modifying your running form by running barefoot or in ultra-minimal shoes, you should be aware that though some changes may occur instantly, progressive change may continue to occur over a long period of time. Just how long it might take can be difficult to predict, and patience is therefore critical. As we have seen, rapid changes can exceed the body's ability to adapt, and pushing form change too hard in a new pair of shoes (or barefoot) might just land you in a doctor's office!

Does Foot Strike Type Even Matter?

If foot strike patterns are variable, and the specific interaction between the foot and the ground is influenced by multiple factors like speed, surface, and footwear, it shouldn't come as a surprise that there's a general lack of consensus on just what one's feet should be doing while one is running. Thus the obvious question arises: "Does foot strike type even matter?"

Each foot comes into contact with the ground some 80 to 100 times per minute on average—this translates to a stride rate or cadence of 160 to 200 steps per minute, with considerable variation from person to person, and at different running speeds. Every time you land, your foot impacts the ground with a certain amount of force, which is counteracted by an equal and opposite amount of force applied by the ground to your foot. This equal and opposite force is known as the ground reaction force, or GRF for short. The ground reaction force comes in a number of components, typically broken into anterior-posterior (along the direction you are traveling), horizontal (side-to-side), and vertical (straight up and down). Of these, the vertical GRF is the greatest in magnitude, and is the one we will focus on here.

The graph below depicts a hypothetical vertical ground reaction force curve for a heel striking barefoot runner (Figure 7-5):

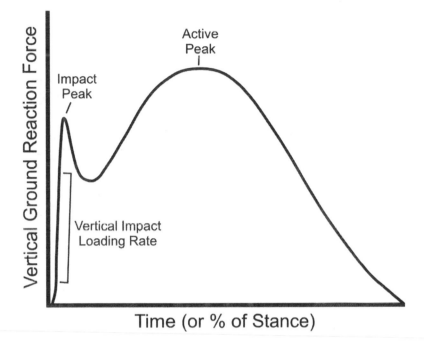

Figure 7-5. Hypothetical vertical ground reaction force plot for a barefoot heel strike.

On the vertical (Y) axis is the value of the vertical ground reaction force as a function of body weight. You can think of the vertical ground reaction force as the amount of force that each collision with the ground exerts directly upward through your foot. The horizontal (X) axis shows time in milliseconds—the amount of time each foot is in contact with the ground varies among people and at different running speeds, but 300 milliseconds (about ⅓ of a second) is a reasonable estimate for a typical recreational runner. The curve depicted on the graph shows how vertical GRF changes from the point of initial contact of the foot with the ground (time 0) to the point where the foot leaves the ground on toe-off (about 300 ms). What you'll notice in this graph is that there are two distinct force peaks. First, the impact peak, sometimes called the passive peak, is the initial reaction force applied by the ground to the foot and lower leg at initial heel contact (remember, this graph is for a heel-toe runner). Full body weight is not being applied at this point, so the impact peak is basically a function of the weight of some portion of the foot and lower leg hitting the ground. The active peak is a function of the force applied by the foot and supported body weight during roughly mid-stance. Notice that it is larger and longer in duration than the impact peak.

In Figure 7-5, vertical loading rate is the slope of the line from initial contact to the impact peak (in practice, it is usually measured in the region from 20 to 80 percent between these points). The loading rate simply represents how quickly the impact force is applied—a steeper slope means a more rapid collision. A more gentle slope would indicate that force application during impact is being spread out over a longer period of time. A reasonable analogy would be punching the wall with your bare fist—your fist comes to a very rapid stop and the force is applied quickly. This is not a good thing for your fist! On the other hand, if you put on a boxing glove, you could still hit the wall really hard, but the cushion in the glove would slow down the impact and distribute the force over a longer period of time. Consequently, it would not hurt as much, and would likely not damage the bones in your hand. The same logic applies to crumple zones in a car—in a crash the crumple zone slows down force application to protect the driver and passengers from the sudden shock of an immediate impact.

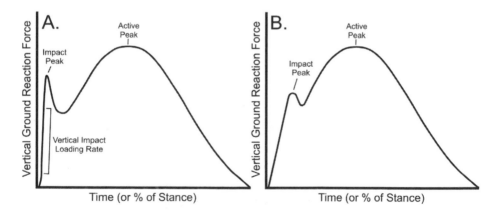

Figure 7-6. Hypothetical vertical ground reaction force plots for a barefoot heel strike (**A.**) and for a heel strike in a shoe with a cushioned sole (**B.**). Note the reduction in height of the impact peak and the reduced vertical impact loading rate in plot B.

Because loading rate increases dramatically, and along with it the risk of an injury like a stress fracture, heel striking while running barefoot is probably not a sustainable option for the long term. Thus, if you are going to run in a heel-toe style, putting cushion under the heel makes perfect sense—it will slow down impact and decrease the loading rate by spreading impact force over a longer period of time (see Figure 7-6). This is a good thing for the heel bone (the calcaneus) and is why many barefoot runners and people who prefer barefoot-style shoes tend to move away from a pronounced heel strike, particularly on hard surfaces (it may not happen instantly, but most will likely adapt with time). The fatty heel pad does not provide enough protection to absorb continual hard impact during barefoot heel-toe running, so your options are either to alter your form or provide some type of protection for your heel.

Now, let's take a look at what usually happens if a runner was to switch to a barefoot forefoot strike (Figure 7-7):

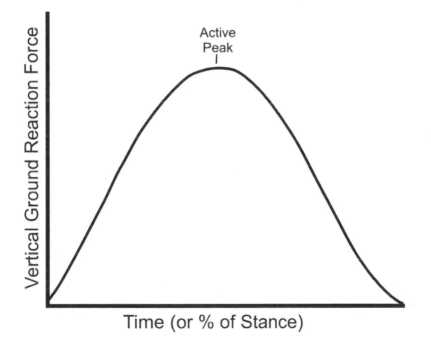

Figure 7-7. Hypothetical vertical ground reaction force plot for a barefoot forefoot strike. Note the absence of the impact peak.

What you'll note is that the distinct impact peak (sometimes referred to as the "impact transient") is now gone. By eliminating the heel strike, the runner has eliminated the impact peak, and the initial slope of the rising force is now lower—loading rate has decreased. The reason for these changes is that instead of absorbing impact via a collision between the heel and the ground, the runner now uses the springiness of the arch of the foot and the Achilles tendon/calf muscle complex to cushion the blow.

Jay Dicharry uses an analogy from the automotive world to illustrate the difference between heel-striking and forefoot striking. If a standard car is like a heel striker, then a monster truck is like a forefoot striker: "Imagine that your car has one shock absorber per axle/per wheel. That shock absorber is there to dissipate a certain amount of stress. Now consider those giant Bigfoot-like monster trucks. These trucks have all of these extra shocks and struts that dissipate the huge amounts of force that those chassis have to endure. If you have more shocks the vehicle can dissipate more load a little bit more evenly and a little bit easier. There's less stress to the system."

"So when you run," continues Dicharry, "if you land with a very prominent, heel strike, the ankle doesn't really give a whole lot. It's a stiff system. So all of the compliance has to be shifted to the knee. And if you do land on the forefoot, what you essentially wind up doing is adding a shock absorber to your chassis. It allows you another joint through which you can dissipate some force." What a forefoot landing also does, though, is add stress to the foot and ankle that a heel striker who is attempting to alter foot strike is likely not adapted to, which could explain the incidence of transition injuries among fledgling barefoot and minimalist runners.

Even though differences in patterns of force application among the different foot strike types do seem to be fairly consistent, Dicharry is careful to point out that foot strike is just one part of overall running form, and that some people do exhibit high impact with a forefoot strike, while others exhibit low impact with a heel strike. "Just because you put somebody on the forefoot doesn't necessarily make everything beautiful, but it is a tool you have available to make a difference."

It's important to highlight that inserting cushioning into shoes to manage impact does work—heel-toe running in a shoe with a cushioned heel does reduce impact loading rate. In fact, Lieberman's barefoot running study showed that average impact loading rate was not significantly different between shod heel-toe runners and barefoot forefoot strikers. As always, it's important to note that variation among individuals was considerable. Lieberman reported that for "the majority of barefoot FFS (forefoot strike) runners, rates of loading were approximately half those of shod RFS (rear foot strike) runners." But even if the cushioned heel reduces impact loading rate so that it's on average equivalent to a barefoot forefoot strike, the foot and leg are generally not positioned the same way in the two conditions. As a result, external forces of similar magnitude can be applied to the body in different ways, and they might be ways that the human body has not evolved to handle as well. Unfortunately, it is quite difficult in practice to know just how the impact reaction force applied by the ground might manifest itself at the level of individual tissues and joints. Though scientists can and do use complex biomechanical models to estimate these forces, to obtain true measures of forces inside or around the ankle, knee, or hip would require implanting sensors into the legs of actual runners—good luck trying to find volunteers for that study!

Why do impact characteristics even matter? There is much debate regarding the potential likelihood of a causal relationship between impact loading rate and running injuries. For example, several studies have linked higher vertical impact loading rates, but not impact peaks, to injuries like lower extremity stress fractures and plantar fasciitis. Additionally, a 2012 study by Adam Daoud, a former student in Daniel Lieberman's lab, shows that Harvard cross-country runners "who habitually rearfoot strike had approximately twice the rate of repetitive stress injuries than individuals who habitually forefoot strike." Conversely, Benno Nigg writes in his book *Biomechanics of Sports Shoes* that based on his research, he feels that "impact forces are not responsible for the development of specific injuries." He points out that internal joint forces at impact are much smaller than they are during the mid-stance phase of the gait cycle when the entire weight of the body bears down on the lower limb. Nigg concludes that "from an impact perspective, the 'cushioning' aspect of shoes needs not take injuries into account." In other words, if the goal is to design shoes to minimize injury risk, they should be designed to manage forces at midstance, not at impact.

Others experts take a more balanced viewpoint, and recognize that both elevated impact and mid-stance forces could be problematic, likely for different types of injuries. For example, based upon his combined clinical and research experience, Jay Dicharry thinks that reducing load-ing rate is critical. "Imagine running fifty miles a week. Think of the amount of wear and tear that occurs on the body," he wrote on his *UVA Endurosport* blog. "Now imagine running fifty miles a week with a gait pattern that causes the mechanical loading of the body to occur less quickly. Decreasing the loading rate applied to tissues will minimize tis-sue stress to the runner, minimizing the effects of the micro-trauma of endurance training." But, like Nigg, Dicharry points out that mid-stance forces are indeed significantly higher and are also extremely important to consider when it comes to injury risk. Given our current state of knowl-edge, forces at both initial impact and at midstance should be considered when it comes to designing running shoes and making recommendations about proper form. A single-minded focus on just one or the other is likely misguided.

Concluding Thoughts and Recommendations

The debate about the relationship between foot-strike type and injury risk is far from over. There are strong opinions all around, and research is ongoing. Among those researchers who do believe that impact-loading rate is linked to injury, their interest tends to focus on whether impact management is better accomplished by heel-toe running in cushioned shoes with a raised heel, or barefoot-style running with a midfoot or fore-foot strike in minimal shoes or no shoes at all. Firm conclusions remain elusive, and perhaps the best advice we can offer to distance runners is the following: On one end of the spectrum, avoid an extreme heel strike (think 45 degree angle between shoe sole and ground at contact); and on the other end, running up on your toes and not letting your heel touch down is also unwise.

Yet despite recent demonization of the heel strike, it's worth mention-ing this observation gleaned from watching race footage of Abebe Bikila. The barefoot 1960 Rome Olympic marathon champion was a mild heel-striker when he won the 1964 Tokyo Olympic Marathon in Puma shoes. Furthermore, today's elites can be observed using all three types of foot strike. Thus, it's quite possible that Bill Bowerman was right back in 1967 when he stated that there is ". . . no one method that you must use. Study each and choose the one that is most comfortable, efficient and works best for you."

So is there even a "one-footstrike-fits-all" scenario? Daniel Lieberman says no, expressing skepticism that there exists one optimal type of foot strike that should be used under all conditions. "I think everybody does everything. This idea that you're just a forefoot striker, or just a midfoot striker, or just a heel striker is bizarre. Variation is what biology is all about—everybody does everything! I think barefoot runners heel strike sometimes, of course they do. I don't think they do it all the time. It's speed dependent, terrain dependent, warm up dependent, etc."

Lieberman even recognizes the importance of variability in his own running, saying "sometimes I go barefoot, sometimes I wear shoes, sometimes I heel strike, sometimes I forefoot strike. Why do people have to do just one thing?"

Precisely.

Perhaps the most prudent advice when it comes to the running foot strike is that if you are not injured, maintain the status quo—don't mess with success! However, if you are experiencing chronic running-related injuries, it might be worth attempting something different. Forces and their application to the body clearly change in some ways with changes in foot strike, and modifying foot strike is one (but not the only) tool that can be used in an attempt to resolve problems. If you do make a change, be aware that it will likely feel very strange at first, and try to not obsess too much about what your feet are doing; overcompensation for a perceived form flaw can be just as problematic as the flaw was to begin with. (For example, running way up on your toes because you heard humans are supposed to forefoot strike). There's no need to rush change, and no need to emulate a form that might not be ideal for your individual body—experiment and find what works, but don't force anything.

⌘

CHAPTER 8

⌒∞⌒

The Running Stride

Running while skipping rope is a great form drill; you can't overstride!

—MARK CUCUZZELLA, M.D.

Runners are obsessed with their feet. They agonize about buying the right kind of running shoes, while habitually scrutinizing the wear patterns on their shoe soles, looking for tell-tale signs that something might not be quite right with their foot strike. It's this concern with foot striking that has made it one of the hottest topics in the current running form debate; but the reality is that the foot strike represents only a single aspect of one's overall running gait, and it might not even be the most important.

It's critical to remember that the foot can't be looked at in isolation from the rest of the body; it's connected to the leg, the legs are connected to the hips, the hips are connected to the vertebral column, and the vertebrae are connected to the head. All of the bones in these structures are linked together by ligaments, muscles and tendons, creating one big, interconnected chain where activity at one location can both influence, and be affected by, activity at any other. Got a pain in your knee? Well, the origin of that pain may have nothing to do with the knee itself, but might rather stem from an issue somewhere higher or lower in the chain (for example, the hips or the foot).

And let's not forget your hands and arms! What you do with them can affect the torso, whose movements rotate the trunk, which can in turn influence what your legs are doing down below while you run. All of these structures function together to assist in your forward motion, and the coordinated whole must function properly should you want to move efficiently and injury free.

In this chapter we examine the running stride. Our approach once again is to start by addressing how the shod human running stride differs from that of the barefoot runner (and by proxy our unshod ancestors), and then to consider whether any of the differences observed might play a causal role in the epidemic of overuse injuries that plague contemporary running.

The Barefoot Difference

Multiple studies have attempted to document the biomechanical differences between barefoot and shod running strides. Unfortunately, it's difficult to know if these studies provide useful information about what runners do when outside of a controlled laboratory environment. Is running on a treadmill a good simulation of running on the road? Is the gait of a shod runner who runs with his or her shoes off for the first time really representative of that of a seasoned barefoot runner? Is a study that looks at runners who pass by a camera or over a force-recording platform along a short indoor runway particularly relevant when compared to real-world running? Do any of these methodologies provide information about what a runner might look like on a mountain trail or at mile twenty of a marathon? All of these are valid questions, and must be kept in mind when interpreting existing scientific studies of running mechanics. Given these issues, as well as the widely varying methodological approaches employed by different researchers, results of published studies that have compared barefoot and shod running are sometimes contradictory. Nonetheless, some general trends or characteristics have been identified among barefoot runners as compared to runners in shoes.

- The foot is more plantarflexed (angled downward) prior to ground contact, and initial contact is more likely to be at the midfoot or fore-foot.
- The ankle goes through a greater range of motion after contact is made.
- The knee tends to be more flexed at initial ground contact, but tends to go through less total range of motion.
- The shin tends to be oriented more vertically at initial ground contact.
- Peak pressures under the heel, midfoot, and big toe are lower
- The calf muscles show greater pre-activation in preparation for landing.
- Stride length decreases.
- Stride rate increases.
- Flight time, the amount of time both feet are in the air, is shorter.
- Vertical impact force is reduced.
- The rate of impact force application (loading rate) is similar to that seen in shod heel strikers, but is applied and absorbed in a different way. Instead of at the heel, impact in barefoot runners is typically applied at the forefoot and absorbed by the Achilles tendon and calf muscles.

To summarize then, barefoot runners tend to avoid or minimize heel striking; they take shorter, quicker strides; they bend the knee more at contact; and the stride is less impactful. On the other hand, runners in shoes tend to heel strike; they take longer, slower strides; they land with a straighter leg; and they generate greater impact when the foot strikes the ground. Though it's fairly easy to identify distinctions like these that emerge in a research environment, it's far more challenging to understand the significance of these differences or to provide advice to runners based upon these findings.

However, there's indeed a degree of certainty that shoes change how we run—they encourage us to run in a way that is quite different than the form likely exhibited by our unshod ancestors. Whether these changes are for the better or for the worse remains an open question, and it is a topic that continues to be hotly debated by runners, coaches, biomechanical researchers, and health care professionals. With that said, let's take a more detailed look at the human running stride and attempt to address the significance of some of the differences observed.

The Running Stride

From a biomechanical standpoint, a running "stride" is defined as the distance from the contact point of one foot to the next contact point of the same foot. In other words, a full stride incorporates three "foot-meets-ground" contacts—left-right-left, or right-left-right. A running stride consists of two major phases:

1. Stance Phase—the period of time during which the foot of one leg is in contact with the ground. Stance begins at initial foot contact with the ground and ends at toe-off.
2. Swing Phase—the period of time during which the leg swings through the air in preparation for the next landing. Swing begins at toe-off and ends with the next ground contact of the swing foot.

   In contrast, a running "step" is the distance between two successive "foot-meets-ground" contacts. In this case, it's right-left, or left-right, and is a function of the following:

1. How far the foot (and leg) that is initially in contact with the ground trails behind the body prior to toe-off.
2. The distance covered during a double-flight phase in which a runner is propelled through the air with neither foot in contact with the ground.
3. How far in front of the body the opposite leg makes contact with the ground during landing.

   From a practical standpoint, stride length and stride rate (number of strides taken per minute; also known as cadence) are important because they are the two determinants of running speed—increase or decrease either while holding the other constant and you will run faster or slower. Similarly, a fixed speed can be maintained with varying combinations of stride rate and length. If you observe ten people running at the same pace, some will probably have short strides and a rapid cadence, and others will have longer strides and a slower cadence. Furthermore, as discussed above, stride rate and stride length are two of the variables that are consistently found to differ between barefoot and shod runners—barefooters tend to take shorter, quicker strides, whereas shod runners usually take longer, slower strides.

The big, looming questions for runners are how these varying stride rate and stride length combinations affect efficiency, and whether the specific combination employed might exhibit a relationship to injury risk. As with almost every topic in the running world, opinions and advice abound, and optimal stride rate and stride length are among the most often discussed and debated aspects of running form. Should we run like the *Looney Tunes* Road Runner, legs spinning rapidly under our body, or should we run with a long, loping stride in order to maximize the ground covered with each step? In contrast with foot-strike types, there appears to be greater agreement concerning the stride: the excessively long-striding or overstriding runner tends to be less efficient, and places himself or herself at increased risk for injury.

Overstriding

When it comes to running, a long stride is often regarded as a thing of beauty. In his 1908 training manual titled *Running and Cross-Country Running*, the great British middle-distance runner Alfred Shrubb commented on this tendency, saying "Critics talk and write enthusiastically on 'long, springing' strides, of men who 'move freely from their hips,' and whose magnificently free action simply devours the ground. These critics mean well, no doubt, but they don't do long-distance running any good." Shrubb goes on to explain his reason for being critical: "For however pretty this stylish running may look, it speedily brings on leg-weariness. A man who 'throws out' his foreleg is bound to tire his knee-joints, while the man who strides high and long . . . will in the long run cover less ground at a greater exertion than the man who lifts his feet and body clear from the track for as short a while and as little as possible. A high, springing stride inevitably means a jarring return to earth, to say nothing of a straining of the joints employed."

Shrubb, who set multiple distance-running world records despite having a stride that was referred to in his own book as "the most ugly in existence," was not the only running great from the past to come down hard on the long stride. In his 1935 book titled *Running*, South African ultrarunner Arthur Newton, who often averaged 200 miles per week, wrote that "Every single way you look at it the long stride for a long journey is wrong. . . . The further you step, the further apart become the points where you are supported by your feet against the action of gravitation . . . the longer your stride the more you bob up and down while employing it . . . you must try to avoid excessive action of this sort as far as possible, as it means that you are using a whole lot of muscles and energy which are not in any way helping you along."

It might be tempting to dismiss the writings of these old-time runners as nothing more than historical curiosities—after all, their records have now been eclipsed by runners employing modern-training techniques. However, opposition to the excessively long stride is still common today. For example, the "magic" number of 180 steps per minute is often thrown around these days as being the optimal cadence for a runner, with the implication being that most runners run with a step rate that is too low and thus a stride length that is too long (more on this in a bit). Similarly, one often hears that runners should shorten their stride by aiming to land directly under their center of mass. We'll ignore for a moment the fact that there is no concrete evidence that 180 is optimal, and that landing directly under your center of mass is in most cases impossible, and instead consider what these oft-repeated nuggets of advice are attempting to correct: overstriding. Among the many things a runner can do wrong with their gait, overstriding is perceived almost universally to be one of the worst when it comes to both injury risk and running efficiency, and it is one of the most commonly observed gait flaws in the modern, shod runner.

Although it has been somewhat variably defined, the term "overstride" is generally applied in reference to the landing phase of running, and describes when ground contact occurs too far out in front of the center of mass of the body. The phrase "center of mass," sometimes used interchangeably with "center of gravity," is frequently stated in the running literature, both popular and scientific, and refers to the average location of the mass or weight of an object. For example, if you were to try to balance a pencil perpendicularly across your extended finger, the location where you could balance it evenly without it falling off would be the center of mass of the pencil. In a human standing vertically, the center of mass is located somewhere along the midline of the body extending from the head through the feet—functionally, it's located roughly in the region of the hips. If you were to lean forward from the ankles while keeping your legs straight and feet planted firmly on the ground, your center of mass would move forward as well. Lean too far forward, and gravity acting vertically downward through your center of mass will cause you to topple over (note: gravity is a vertical force and will not pull you forward as suggested by some running-form schools).

Determining when a runner is landing too far in front of his or her center of mass is difficult in practice—how far is too far? As such, a more practical definition of overstriding is as follows: overstriding is when a runner reaches out excessively with the foot and lower leg such that at ground contact the ankle lands in front of a line drawn vertically through the knee (see Figure 8-1). The farther in front of the knee that the ankle falls, the greater the overstride.

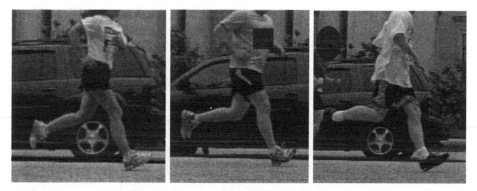

Figure 8-1. Images of representative overstriding runners taken from a high-speed video recording of a 5-kilometer road race. All images represent the moment of initial contact between the foot and the ground—note that the ankle is well ahead of the knee in all three images.

Definitions based on forward reaching of the lead leg have been applied for decades. For example, Fred Wilt, a two-time Olympian (1948 and 1952 in the 10,000 meters) and former coach of the Purdue University women's track and cross-country teams, wrote the following in his 1964 book *Run Run Run*: "The leading leg should never be stretched forward in an exaggerated effort to achieve a longer stride." In their 1967 book *Jogging*, Bill Bowerman and W. E. Harris also advise against overstriding, writing that "Each foot falls just under the knee. Don't reach out with the foot and overstride." Similarly, Dr. George Sheehan asked the following question as part of his overuse syndrome "systems analysis" in his 1978 book *Medical Advice for Runners*: "Are you landing properly, with the knee bent and the foot never getting in front of the knee?" Unfortunately for many recreational runners, and even some elites, the answer to Sheehan's question is all too often "no."

Adding more complexity to his recommendation, Bowerman elaborated on overstriding and his vision of proper running form in an article from a 1971 issue of *Sports Illustrated* titled "The Secrets of Speed":

> *When your foot first makes contact with the ground two fundamentals must be carefully observed. First, your foot should strike after it has reached its farthest point of advance and has actually started to swing back. Second, when your foot first strikes, the point of contact should be directly under your knee, not out in front of it, and as nearly as possible squarely beneath your center of gravity. Fortunately, both fundamentals are easy enough to comply with by keeping your knees slightly bent at all times and by not overstriding. If the foot hits the ground ahead of the knee, the leg will be too straight and will act as a brake instead of an accelerator. The entire body will be severely jolted with each stride. This creates fatigue, pain, and possibly eventual injury.*

Bowerman covers lots of ground in this *Sports Illustrated* excerpt. He says that overstriding is bad, that it increases braking forces, that it jolts the legs and can increase injury risk. Hence, a runner should strive to land as close to directly underneath the center of mass as possible, and that the aim is to strike the ground after the foot has reached its farthest point of advance. Almost forty years later, running journalist and author Scott Douglas makes many of the same points in a 2010 issue of *Running Times*:

> *Overstriding means that your feet land significantly in front of your center of gravity. When this happens, you're unable to make full use of your fitness, because you're braking with every step. And you might soon be breaking with every step, in that overstriding amplifies the already-strong impact forces of running and therefore can contribute to more strain on your bones, muscles, and ligaments.*

Apparently, many runners have not gotten the message. In slow-motion video clips of typical non-elite runners in a race, it's quite common to observe people landing with nearly straight legs, feet extended well in front of the knee, and a foot that is angled upward toward the sky. Furthermore, many runners violate Bowerman's directive to not let the foot contact the ground before the lower leg has finished its forward swing—in fact, some runners, particularly when fatigued, will actually skid forward into a landing. (If you have extensive wear on the outer-rear margin of your shoes, you might be a scuffer of this sort.)

So how is it that after more than 100 years of athletes, coaches, and writers shouting warnings about the risks of overstriding, this nettlesome gait flaw is still so prevalent in just about any road race? Part of the reason, one can certainly suspect, is running shoes. For the past several decades, running shoes have been designed for the specific purpose of reducing impact, which is a major outcome of overstriding. Quite rightly, runners who overstride and pound the ground with their heels need cushioning under the rear portion of the foot. As a result, heel cushioning has become more elaborate, and cushioning "technology" in the heel requires space that has necessitated that heels become even larger still. And herein lies the problem—the rear portion of the sole of a shoe with a 12mm cushioning differential between the heel and forefoot extends both far below and typically well behind the actual heel of the foot. This particular footwear construction virtually guarantees that contact characteristics will differ from barefoot running because there is simply more shoe to get in the way of a runner's natural stride.

Following Bill Bowerman's advice to contact the ground after the leg has started to swing back is difficult in shoes with a large, cushioned heel because the heel can catch the ground before swing-back can even begin; and once the heel catches it forces the forefoot to slap downward as the foot is torqued about the ankle. As the cushioned heel gets larger and larger (for example, by adding springs or other gratuitous "impact absorbing" gadgets), it's probably even more likely that a runner will overstride. It's a vicious cycle where the overstride calls for cushion, and cushion allows the overstride to become even more pronounced, to the point where it is hard to avoid. Just as Peter Cavanagh suggested back in 1980 that thickening of the cushioned heel of running shoes might have contributed to rearfoot instability and thus the rise of pronation control technology, raising the heel might also be encouraging a more impactful gait, necessitating ever larger amounts of cushion. In other words, modern running shoes may be creating problems that require "more shoe" to correct. It's a catch-22.

Dr. Steven Robbins, an M.D. and associate professor of mechanical engineering at Concordia University in Montreal, has written extensively on the effects of cushioning and footwear on running gait, and in a series of papers from the late 1980's and early 1990's he outlined a number of mechanisms by which running shoes alter one's stride. He summarized many of these points in a 1990 article in the journal *Sports Medicine*.

Robbins suggested that an extremely soft, cushioned running shoe encourages pre-emptive stiffening of the leg prior to landing as a runner searches for stability and attempts to prevent the foot from rolling inward or outward on the compressible sole after contact is made. In other words, running in a soft, cushioned shoe causes you to tense certain of your leg muscles in preparation for landing since you know your foot is about to collide with an unstable surface. This response is similar to how your body reacts to running on surfaces of varying hardness—the softer the surface, the more you stiffen your legs when your foot lands (try running on gym mats or a trampoline and see what happens). This response could in part explain why runners in heavily cushioned shoes tend to both land on their heels and have straighter legs at contact. In support of this hypothesis, a study published in 2003 in the *Journal of Biomechanics* by Vinzenz von Tscharner and colleagues from the University of Calgary demonstrated that shod runners exhibit more intense preactivation (or pre-firing) of the tibialis anterior muscle on the front of the shin prior to ground contact than barefoot runners—this muscle is responsible for lifting the front portion of the foot up (dorsiflexion) prior to a heel strike. Altering what is on your feet thus changes the action of your muscles, and these changes are initiated before the foot even contacts the ground.

In addition to creating instability by putting a soft landing surface under the foot, Robbins emphasized that shoe soles rob your feet of critical sensory input from the ground surface, and he believes that this can have a dramatic effect on running form. For example, he thinks that one will modify the interaction between the foot and the ground in order to minimize painful sensations caused by surface irregularity or the presence of ground debris like pebbles or sharp twigs. As anyone who has tried to run barefoot on asphalt or concrete knows firsthand, initial attempts (depending on distance) will often result in serious blistering of the skin on the bottoms of the feet. Some of this might be due to a lack of conditioning (the bare skin is simply too tender, especially if one has been wearing shoes since childhood). But the skin abrasion that occurs might also be caused by a lack of behavioral adaptation. Robbins indicates that due to the highly sensory nature of the soles of the human feet, barefoot runners learn to avoid shearing between the foot and the ground by adapting their stride to minimize friction. Repeatedly skidding forward into a landing would be quite damaging for a barefoot runner! What many barefoot runners tend to do instead is land just as described by Bowerman—after the foot has reached its forward-most swing or even after it has just started to come back. In watching slow-motion videos of barefoot runners on asphalt, it often seems as if the foot pauses in the air for a split second just before it touches down—it's as if the foot is waiting for its forward velocity to match that of the rest of the body before contacting the rough surface below. A good way to visualize this is to think about the motion of the foot when propelling a scooter or skateboard—you don't want it to first plow forward into the ground, then reverse direction and start pushing. The friction generated might not hurt if you're wearing shoes, but you can be sure that doing it regularly would rapidly wear down the sole.

If Robbins is correct, then the form adaptations made by barefoot runners are not geared solely toward managing impact, but also include protective mechanisms aimed at preventing damage to the skin on the sole of the foot. Putting on shoes of any type (even the most minimal) removes the need for this protective response, and this could explain why running form of barefoot runners changes in certain noticeable ways— longer stride, reduced cadence, longer flight phase—even when they put on ultra-minimal shoes like the Vibram FiveFingers. Even though there are now plenty of new barefoot-style and minimalist shoes without much or any cushion, making a shoe that allows similar plantar sensation as going completely barefoot is simply not possible. Furthermore, any protective covering on the sole, no matter how thin, is going to dramatically reduce friction between the skin and ground. As a result, it is quite unlikely that any form of footwear will perfectly replicate what it is like to run barefoot.

Consider the irony: Bill Bowerman, who was a co-founder of Nike, advocated that runners should avoid doing all of the things that modern cushioned shoes with beefed-up heels encouraged them to do with their form. The ideal form, he maintained, is instead more typical of speedy elites and those who regularly run barefoot. Although the straight-legged heel strike is common among shod runners, unless you're running on an exceedingly soft surface (such as sand), it's not something you would likely do for any length of time if you were barefoot. Though some barefoot runners do in fact heel strike, and some do overstride with a forefoot strike (overstriding can occur with any type of foot strike, and a forefoot overstride can be just as problematic), it's extremely rare to see a barefoot runner who combines a pronounced overstride with a significant heel strike—to do so would be far too jarring on the heel bone and lower leg. The combination of overstriding and a massive heel strike seems to be a modern phenomenon, and it might just be that this unnatural pairing is causing us harm.

Is Overstriding Bad?

It's all well and good to posit that gait adaptations caused by shoes might be a cause of some running injuries, but speculation should not be the basis upon which runners decide to ditch their shoes or modify their stride. A better approach is to consider the evidence that suggests that overstriding and related gait characteristics are in fact problematic, and to then explore approaches to overcoming the overstride.

Let's take a look at two studies that support the notion that longer strides increase joint loading, and thus might increase injury risk:

Stride Study #1

A 1998 article in the journal *Medicine and Science in Sports and Exercise* discusses in depth the relationship between stride length and impact absorption in running. The authors of the article, lead by Dr. Timothy Derrick from Iowa State University, point out that when a runner's foot makes initial contact with the ground during the landing phase of the gait cycle, the body rapidly decelerates during the collision, and a shock wave is transmitted through the body. Because it is imperative to keep the head stable in order to maintain the ability to see straight and prevent the brain from rattling around in the skull, the body has built-in mechanisms that attenuate or diminish the magnitude of this shock wave before it reaches the head.

Shock-dissipating structures in the human body include the bones and cartilage in the feet, legs, hips, and vertebral column, and the muscles and tendons that attach to your skeleton. Because of both their elasticity and their ability to adapt contraction strength to the demands of the situation, your muscles are the most effective shock absorbers. As impact is applied at the foot and your joints begin bend, the muscles around the rotating joints are tensed in order to prevent each joint from collapsing. In this process, they "absorb" some of the impact energy. This is why you aim to land with bent legs rather than straight legs when jumping down from a height—better to brace your fall with your leg muscles rather than your leg bones. A straight-legged landing is far more likely to be jaw-jarring and teeth-rattling!

Derrick and his colleagues' goal with their experiment was to determine how decreasing and increasing stride length from a runner's naturally chosen value at a given speed might affect impact energy absorption and thus shock attenuation at the ankle, knee, and hip. In other words, could an alteration of stride length affect how one manages the impact shock wave as it races from the feet up to the head, and if so, what implications might this have for injury risk?

To conduct the experiment, the researchers attached shock sensing accelerometers to the shins and foreheads of their subjects—this would allow them to estimate shock dissipation from the lower leg to the skull. Each runner ran across a force plate at his normal, naturally chosen stride length, and then at (plus or minus) 10 percent and (plus or minus) 20 percent of the normal stride length (using longer or shorter strides than he would freely choose). What Derrick's team found was that as stride length increased from normal, shock magnitude increased and progressed further up the body from foot to head—this resulted in increased impact energy absorption by the knee and hip. As stride length decreased, impact energy absorption at all three joints—the hip, knee, and ankle—decreased significantly. Of particular interest is the fact that the specific way impact energy was dissipated by the joints was dependent on stride length. Though all three joints contributed to impact energy absorption while running with a stride 20 percent longer than what was normal for the runners, the long stride placed a disproportionate fraction of the work on the knee, which is the most commonly injured joint in runners. In contrast, when running with a stride 20 percent shorter than normal impact absorption was shared almost equally by the ankle and knee, and the hip contributed very little.

The results of this study indicate that running with a long stride places greater stress on the muscles and connective tissues that support the knees and hips. Not only could this increase risk of overuse injury, it also requires the large muscles around these joints to be more metabolically active. Studies have indeed shown that longer strides are associated with greater energy utilization (and thus reduced efficiency), whereas runners can increase stride rate by as much as 10 percent (and thus shorten their stride) without incurring a metabolic penalty (more on this later). If speed over a short distance is the goal, a long stride may not be a big problem, but over the course of a marathon or an ultra a long stride could be a recipe for disaster.

Stride Study #2

In 2011, Dr. Bryan Heiderscheit, a physical therapist and associate professor in the Department of Orthopedics and Rehabilitation at the University of Wisconsin, published a study with colleagues in the journal *Medicine & Science in Sport & Exercise* that to a degree reproduced but also expanded upon the research done by Derrick's team. Heiderscheit noted that increasing stride rate and thus lowering stride length appears to have positive benefits for joint loading, but that increasing stride rate too much has negative impacts in terms of efficiency. Thus, he conducted a study to look at the effects of more moderate modifications of step rate/length on running mechanics and joint loading, and he looked at loading over a longer period of the stance phase. (Authors' Note: the phrases "step rate" and "stride rate" are sometimes used interchangeably, which can be confusing. Step rate is the number of steps taken per minute; stride rate is the number of strides taken per minute. Since each stride is composed of two steps, step rate is equal to two times stride rate.)

In the Heiderscheit study, forty-five recreational runners ran on a treadmill (each wearing his or her own training shoes) at step rates both 5 percent and 10 percent below (slower cadence) and above (faster cadence) their normal, freely chosen step rate. All trials were run at the same speed (a "moderate intensity" pace chosen by each individual). They concurrently measured forces underfoot, and made a variety of biomechanical measurements of the runners at the various step rates.

With a step rate increase of only 5 percent relative to the naturally chosen step rate, this is what the study found:

1. Reduced loading of the knee.
2. Reduced step length.
3. Shifted the initial point of contact between the foot and the ground so that the foot landed closer to the body.
4. Reduced braking forces.
5. Reduced the vertical excursion of the center of mass (less up and down movement of the body).
6. Reduced peak adduction angle of the hip (less inward angling of the thigh).
7. Reduced peak flexion angle (bending) of the knee during stance phase.

Heiderscheit's team also found that in addition to the changes listed above, a step rate increase of 10 percent resulted in the following:

1. Reduced loading of the hip.
2. Reduced stance duration.
3. Reduced inclination of the foot at initial ground contact (less pronounced heel strike).
4. Reduced peak vertical ground reaction force.
5. Increased rating of perceived exertion (runners felt they were working harder).
6. Reduced peak flexion angle of the hip.
7. Reduced peak hip abduction torque.
8. Reduced peak hip internal rotation torque.
9. Increased knee flexion angle at initial ground contact.
10. Reduced peak knee extension torque.

Generally speaking, most of the above variables changed in the opposite direction when step rate was decreased by 5 or 10 percent, and somewhat surprisingly, the ankle only showed increased loading when step rate was reduced by 10 percent from normal. Thus, running with shorter, quicker steps tended to reduce joint loading, whereas longer, slower steps increased loading of all three of the major joints in the leg.

Looking at these results, it seems like running with shorter, quicker steps provides much positive benefit with little negative consequence beyond a slightly greater perceived exertion if step rate is increased by 10 percent from what is normal for that runner. One notices that loading of joints is reduced, braking force and up/down movement are reduced (both of which can be linked to improved efficiency), and several biomechanical measures associated with injuries are lessened. As an example of the latter, Heiderscheit writes that excessive hip adduction and internal rotation have been associated with knee injuries and iliotibial band syndrome, and suggests that "running with a step rate greater than preferred . . . may be useful in the clinical management of running injuries involving the hip."

The Heiderscheit study concludes that "subtle changes in step rate can reduce the energy absorption required of the lower extremity joints, which may prove beneficial in the prevention and treatment of running injuries," and that the "knee joint appeared to be most sensitive to changes in step rate." Furthermore, the authors highlighted that "many of the biomechanical changes we found when step rate increased are similar to those observed when running barefoot or with minimalist footwear."

On the *Runner's World Peak Performance* blog, Amby Burfoot interviewed Heiderscheit about his study. He asked him what he thought would have happened if his subjects had worn racing flats instead of their training shoes, and Heiderscheit responded that: "I'd guess, and this is just speculation, that they wouldn't run the same as in the training shoes. I think they would have selected a preferred stride rate close to our plus five-percent condition." Burfoot later asks whether "thick, cushioned shoes" encourage runners to take a longer stride, to which Heiderscheit responded that there is lots of variability, but that it "seems like a reasonable conclusion." Furthermore, just as Bill Bowerman emphasized that landing should occur "after (the foot) has reached its farthest point of advance and has actually started to swing back," Heiderscheit also stressed the importance of the final moments before ground contact: "A lot of the big action happens at the very end of the stride. Some people fall forward onto their extended foot, while others begin to reverse their foot action before they put the foot down. Thicker shoes probably encourage runners to fall forward onto them."

What's important to remember in considering the results of studies like those conducted by Derrick and Heiderscheit is that though both empirically observed what appear to be positive changes in association with a shorter, quicker stride, these studies do not answer the question of whether such changes actually reduce injury risk. Heiderscheit was very clear about this in his interview with Burfoot, saying that "We decided against pushing the shorter strides harder at this point because we don't have good injury results yet." But based on his own clinical experience treating injured runners, Heiderscheit did say that "if we shorten their strides, a lot of their problems go away." Thus, there is no guarantee that a shorter stride is a cure all for every running injury or that it will even consistently fix a specific problem like knee pain in every runner who suffers from it. However, the results of these studies do suggest that stride manipulation is a potentially useful tool in the treatment of running injuries, and the positive benefits seem to be accrued by adapting patterns away from those encouraged by the modern running shoe.

Pounding vs. Repetition—Which is Worse?

While increasing stride rate and thus decreasing stride length has been found to reduce loading of the joints, running at a higher cadence requires one to take more steps to cover the same distance. This raises the question of which is more detrimental to the body: a lower impact stride that must be repeated more times over a given distance, or a higher impact stride that can cover that distance with fewer repetitions?

In a 2009 study published in *Medicine and Science in Sport and Exercise* that looked at the risk of stress fracture as it relates to stride length, Dr. Brent Edwards of the University of Illinois at Chicago and colleagues determined that reducing stride length by 10 percent should theoretically reduce the risk of suffering a tibial stress fracture, and that "the benefits of reducing strain with stride length manipulation outweigh the detriments of increased loading cycles associated with a given mileage." Furthermore, the study concluded that "these benefits become more pronounced at higher running mileages." Though more research needs to be done on this topic, initial results support the idea that the load-reducing benefits of increasing stride rate outweigh the risks of having to cycle through a greater number of strides on each run.

On Anecdotes and the Running Stride

Let's temporarily move away from the hard science and address a topic that's certainly less empirical and data-driven: anecdotal evidence. While these "findings" are often dismissed as unscientific, it does not mean that they have little value. Subjective experience is what many of us have to go on. We might like a certain shoe or feel that a technique "cured" a chronic injury. Furthermore, when there's mounting anecdotal evidence about a particular issue or problem, this should be a sign for further study. Brian Heiderscheit told Amby Burfoot that one of the reasons that he conducted his study on stride-rate manipulation was his clinical observation that patients sometimes reported that their knee-injury symptoms improved when they ran faster, and faster running is typically coupled with a higher stride rate and possibly changes in landing characteristics. This is an ideal example of how anecdotal observations can stimulate more detailed scientific study, which in turn can aid in the development of treatment strategies.

Anecdotes have played a big role in fueling the recent barefoot running trend and consumer interest in minimalist footwear. You've probably read about or heard fellow runners claiming that switching to barefoot running or a barefoot-style stride made all of their injuries go away. What they may not reveal is that sometimes new and different injuries do appear (often to bones, muscles, ligaments or tendons associated with the ankles or feet), but let's assume that these individuals are being honest (given the number of these reports, surely some of them are) and relate these anecdotal reports to the science just discussed. As we noted at the beginning of this chapter, one of the major differences that has been consistently observed in comparisons of shod vs. barefoot runners is that the barefooters tend to adopt a shorter, quicker stride. Thus, we might speculate that one of the ways that running barefoot or with barefoot-style form might help some people overcome injury is that it facilitates a change in running gait, and that change alters the way that forces are applied to the joints. The studies by Derrick and Heiderscheit provide plausible mechanisms by which this might occur—running with a shorter, quicker stride seems to take some of the load off the knees and hips, so those suffering from injuries associated with these joints may experience relief when their stride shortens up even just a small amount.

The next step in the process of scientific investigation is to actually put stride length modification as a treatment strategy to the test—try it out on a group of injured runners and see what happens. According to an August 2010 article by Alex Hutchinson in the *Globe and Mail*, Heiderscheit has been doing just that by conducting a trial that compares stride rate modification to standard care for the treatment of knee pain and iliotibial band syndrome. It will take awhile for the results to fully materialize, so it's currently up to each runner and therapist to individually decide whether they find existing evidence of benefit sufficient, or whether it's better to wait for concrete results on injury outcomes. For the perennially injured runner who has nothing to lose though, doing a bit of experimentation with form or footwear either on his or her own or under the guidance of a coach or physical therapist seems like an easy choice—when the alternative is not running at all or being miserable when you do so, why not try something different?

The Need for Speed

You've probably noticed that we've written little in this book about speed—the omission is intentional. Though running fast may win races and satisfy individual performance goals (who doesn't like setting a new PR), speed increases forces and thus increases injury risk.

"Running to compete" has been identified as a risk factor for injury in runners, and if you make a decision to compete in races and chase time goals, then you must accept that there is some risk associated with doing so. Elite athletes accept this risk every day—to be able to perform their best in competition, they run a very fine line in attempting to maximize the benefits of training without pushing so hard that they get hurt. But, elite athletes are usually paid to train (it's their job), or they are on scholarships. Furthermore, they typically have support networks, trainers, massage therapists, coaches, and so forth to keep their bodies in highly competitive shape. The elite athlete thus has both needs and means that are very different than those of the weekend warrior.

So, for the majority of runners who run for health, fitness, and enjoyment and perhaps like to let loose in the occasional local 5K (and who have never had the opportunity to sit in a cryosauna, or sleep in a high-altitude simulator), what are the best ways to incorporate speed without getting hurt?

First and foremost, speed should be embraced like any other change in training—gradually and progressively. Don't head out to the track and attempt to knock out ten laps at maximum speed on your first time out! Build slowly and learn to feel comfortable using a faster stride. Regarding the latter, be aware that running faster is usually accomplished initially by adopting a longer stride, so avoid the temptation to lengthen stride by reaching out with the lead leg. If you watch elite runners running fast, they typically elongate their stride on the backside by extending their hip more, which results in the foot and leg trailing further behind the body. This can be difficult if you have tight hip flexors or weak glutes/hamstrings (as most of us who sit at a desk all day probably do), so some flexibility and strengthening work might be advisable. Also, avoid the temptation to launch yourself into the air at too high an angle with each stride—excessive vertical movement wastes energy by requiring your muscles to work harder to support your weight as you come back down.

Although there are risks involved, one of the positive benefits of running fast is that it's a great way to fine-tune your stride. Mistakes are more noticeable when you're running at high speed, particularly if you're wearing racing flats or a similar minimal shoe, and speed work will allow you to feel what it's like to run at a higher cadence.

You might consider starting with speed work by just incorporating a bit of faster paced running at the end of your runs (perhaps barefoot on a track infield). If you find that to be of benefit, you can start to explore more intense speed workouts like track intervals. Regardless of what you choose, the same message applies: always be careful.

Is There an Optimal Stride Rate?

Let's say that you know that you're an overstrider—perhaps your running partner has commented on how you thud the ground when you run, or perhaps you spot a race photo of yourself hitting the ground with an extended knee. Suppose you also have a chronic injury history that you suspect might be related to your less-than-ideal gait, or maybe you think that the braking forces that you generate are holding you back from your next PR. How do you fix this?

There is no shortage of available advice and information on how to go about retooling your stride. In fact, form coaches seem to be popping up all over, and there are entire books and DVD series that provide detailed instruction on how to retrain your gait (for example, *Chi Running, Evolution Running, POSE*). Each form approach has its own idiosyncrasies, and a comparison among them or consideration of their relative merits is beyond the scope of this book. Our own personal take is that we all learn differently, and if you think an informational guide or accredited coach might be useful then do a bit of research on the options and go for it! However, there's no reason that form change can't be accomplished on your own if you have the desire and willingness to expend a bit of time and effort.

Should You Attempt to Run Like the Elites?

One approach to learning about good running form is to watch the elites—they run for a living and have spent more time fine-tuning their form than the vast majority of recreational runners. However, a few things should be kept in mind when trying to emulate the form of elite runners.

First, and most obviously, elite runners in a race are running very fast, and form changes with speed. It makes little sense for a recreational runner who puts in most of their miles at an 8:00 or 9:00 per mile pace to attempt to perfectly mimic the gait of an elite 10,000-meter specialist running at a sub-5:00 per mile pace. Most of us would be better off emulating the relaxed form they employ during their victory lap!

Second, form among elite runners is variable. Alberto Salazar, who won the Boston Marathon once and New York City Marathon three times in the early 1980's, was widely believed to have succeeded despite his form rather than because of it. So even elites may not be perfect role models. Should the average runner mimic the head-bob of Paula Radcliff? Probably not, even though she does happen to own the women's marathon world record. Emil Zatopek was one of the greatest distance runners of all time. But here's how *New York Herald Tribune* sports columnist Red Smith described his form: "He ran like a man with a noose around his neck . . . the most frightful horror spectacle since Frankenstein . . . on the verge of strangulation; his hatchet face was crimson; his tongue lolled out." Another newspaper scribe wrote, "He ran as if his next step would be his last." But Zatopek, a three-time gold medalist in the 1952 Helsinki Olympics, had a ready-made answer for his critics: "I shall learn to have a better style once they start judging races according to their beauty. So long as it's a question of speed then my attention will be directed to seeing how fast I can cover the ground."

There are many factors that make elites capable of throwing down times that the rest of us could only dream of—these include inherent aspects of their anatomy and physiology, training background, motivation, mental toughness, VO_2 max, capacity to endure pain, and so on. Form is just one part of the picture when it comes to elite running success, and it may be a very small part.

Taking this a step further, even if we take a group of elites who experts might classify as having "ideal" form, careful examination will reveal variation among them. Some carry their arms high, some carry them low. Some keep their torso upright, some lean forward a bit. Some spend a bit more time with both feet airborne, some stay closer to the ground. Some heel strike, some land on the midfoot, and others land on the forefoot. There are commonalities among elites that may suggest general patterns, but looking at any single elite's running form as a model of absolute perfection that should be copied is a mistake. Running biomechanist Peter Cavanagh made this very point back in 1980 in the book *The Sweet Spot in Time* by John Jerome: "It doesn't work, for instance, to tell the novice to imitate (Bill) Rodgers . . . Running style, or performance in any sport, eventually boils down to the way you adapt to your own anatomy, your own physiology, to the peculiarities of your own body."

The take-away message for all runners is that each of us is unique—and this applies to the recreational runner as well as the elite. Ultimately, the key is finding the best form for your individual body—whether that's the form that lets you run fastest, most efficiently, or with least chance of injury, that decision is up to you.

You have probably heard or read somewhere that the ideal running stride is to land with the foot directly under your center of mass and to run with a cadence of 180—both of these are aimed at reducing stride length and thus correcting an overstriding gait. Is there any evidence to support this advice? Let's start with center of mass. Unless you are accelerating, like say a sprinter coming out of the blocks, you cannot land directly under your center of mass when you run. Says gait expert Jay Dicharry: "At steady state, the foot does (and should) contact in front of the center of mass." The exact distance that the foot lands in front of the hips varies for sure, but it is always out front. Thus, thinking about landing under your center of mass is a great cue to help get your stride to shorten a bit, but it never happens in reality.

Next let's address the "magic 180." It's not uncommon these days to hear people say that a stride rate of 180 steps per minute is optimal. Witness this passage from an article titled "Stride Right" by two-time

Olympic marathoner Ed Eyestone in the September 2011 issue of *Runner's World*:

> Years ago, researchers determined that elite distance runners ran at a rate of about 180 strides per minute. Indeed, eminent exercise physiologist and coach Jack Daniels tallied the stride rate of every runner in every distance event at the 1984 Olympics in Los Angeles. He found that in events longer than 3000 meters, every runner save one had a stride rate of 180. The outlier had a paltry 178.
>
> While it's not easy to overcome biology, you can move closer to the optimum 180 strides per minute—with practice . . .

As Eyestone's passage points out, this number can be traced back to famed coach Dr. Jack Daniels, who in his classic training manual, *Daniels' Running Formula*, published an observation that elite runners at the 1984 Olympics tended to run at a stride rate of 180 *or more* steps/minute. Yet it's worth noting that this is actually not the first time that the number 180 has been mentioned in relation to running cadence—Arthur Newton recommended a 180 cadence in his 1935 book *Running*. Nonetheless, Daniels is generally considered the father of 180. Based on his observations at the Los Angeles Olympics, which included runners competing in events ranging from 800 meters to the marathon, he also found that the rate "doesn't vary much even when they're not running fast" or in events from 3000 meters on up. Conversely, Daniels writes that when he works with new runners, few if any have a stride rate of 180 or more. He suggests that these long, slow striders are at increased risk for injury, and writes that "the slower you take steps, the longer you're in the air, and the longer you're in the air, the higher you displace your body mass and the harder you hit the ground on landing." This occurs because a slow cadence must be compensated for by a longer stride to maintain a given speed (remember: speed = stride rate × stride length). He advocates that runners work on a "shorter, lighter stride," with the end goal being that their running will become more efficient and they will be less prone to impact related injury. Sounds a lot like what Shrubb and Newton were saying back in the first half of the twentieth century, doesn't it!

Unfortunately, Daniels's findings have been misinterpreted by many runners and coaches who steadfastly believe that all runners should aim to run at exactly a 180 cadence at all times. Daniels never took such a rigid position regarding cadence. Indeed, he provides this advice in his book: "We often talk about getting into a good running rhythm, and the one you want to get into is one that involves 180 *or more* {our emphasis} steps per minute." Essentially, Daniels feels that most runners have a cadence that is too slow, and that they would benefit from speeding it up a bit. An inflexible adherence to 180 steps per minute ignores the fact that cadence is known to change with speed and is probably influenced by other factors. What's more, despite the frequency with which the 180-cadence mantra is repeated, there does not even appear to be any evidence that the 180 number is optimal for every person. Rather, the existing evidence suggests that each individual has an optimal cadence range of their own, and that the primary factor that determines optimal cadence is efficiency. Put simply, most runners seem to choose their individual cadence in order to minimize the energy that they expend when they run.

In 1982, Peter Cavanagh and Keith Williams published a classic paper titled "The Effect of Stride Length Variation on Oxygen Uptake During Distance Running" in the journal *Medicine and Science in Sport and Exercise*. Their goal was to determine how a given runner chooses the specific combination of stride rate and stride length that he employs when he runs. The researchers were intrigued by the idea that runners might subconsciously choose these parameters in order to run with a combination that minimizes energy expenditure at a given speed.

In order to test this hypothesis, Canavagh and Williams had ten experienced male runners run on a treadmill at a pace of 7:00 per mile. They had the runners run at their freely chosen stride rate and length, and using this value as a baseline, had them both increase and decrease stride length by 6.7 percent, 13.4 percent, and 20 percent from their freely chosen values (they used a metronome to vary stride rate, which resulted in the desired change in stride length since speed was held constant). During each running session at each stride length, they recorded oxygen consumption as a measure of energy expenditure (standard procedure in studies of this type). In doing so, they were able to observe how energy expenditure changed as stride length was varied above or below the preferred value for each individual. A higher oxygen consumption at a given stride length indicated that a greater amount of energy was being expended (in other words, the runners were less efficient at the experimental pace).

What Cavanagh and Williams found was that the freely chosen combination of stride rate and stride length was indeed the most energy efficient for most of the runners that they looked at. That is, having the runners artificially increase or decrease their stride length caused them to consume more oxygen (use more energy) than when they were allowed to subconsciously choose their own stride length. Viewed in graphical form (Figure 8-2), plotting energy expenditure against stride length yielded a U-shaped curve for each runner, with freely chosen stride length tending to fall right near the bottom of the U, which is the most economical position.

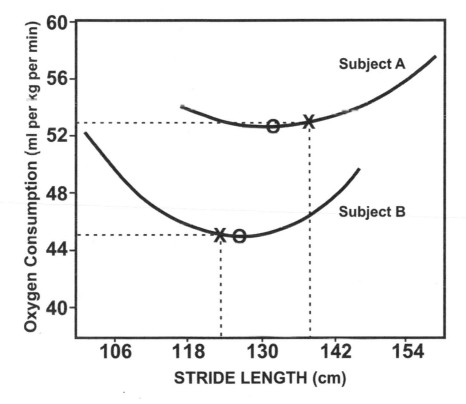

Figure 8-2. Graph adapted from Cavanagh and Williams (1982) showing the relationship between stride length and oxygen consumption (energy expenditure) for two individual subjects. X's indicate normal, freely chosen stride length for each individual, O's indicate optimal stride length for each individual. Note that oxygen consumption at the freely chosen stride length was fairly close to optimal, indicting that the runners tended to run with a stride length that minimized energy expenditure.

In addition to the above relationship, the researchers observed considerable variation among runners in both minimum energy expenditure at the experimental speed, as well as the specific combination of stride rate and stride length employed to minimize energy expenditure. In other words, most runners chose a combination of cadence and stride length that was individually most efficient, but there was no single combination that was most efficient for all of the runners. The upshot of this is that attempting to force all of these individuals to run at the same cadence (for example, 180) would make very little sense.

When looked at on an individual level, the results of Cavanagh and Williams' study yield some interesting findings. For example, they found that the runner with the longest legs had the shortest stride, and that the runner with the shortest legs had among the longest strides. One could imagine a long-legged runner taking short, choppy steps, but how could a short-legged runner come out near the top in a stride length comparison? Details are not provided, but one might possibly suspect that Mr. Shorty was doing some combination of extending the leg behind his body further and generating greater propulsion on takeoff, spending more time in the air during flight phase, or extending the foot farther forward on landing.

When Mr. Long Legs and Mr. Shorty were removed from the study, Cavanagh and Williams still found no strong relationship between leg length and optimal stride length, which indicates that the commonly held belief that longer legged runners take longer strides was not supported by their data. "It is not in general possible to predict optimal stride length in a population on the basis of leg length" writes Cavanagh. This comes as a bit of a surprise since just as individuals of above average height are often assumed to be "born" basketball players, individuals with long legs are often assumed to have a natural advantage when it comes to distance running. The notion that leg length is a poor predictor of stride length has since been supported by additional studies, and thus it's not just a fluke observation of a single experiment. For example, Cavanagh himself did a follow-up study with Rodger Kram, now a biomechanist at the University of Colorado, in a 1989 issue of *Medicine & Science in Sport & Exercise* in which they found only a weak relationship between leg length and stride length. Based upon this result they concluded that "distance running coaches would be unwise to attempt any intervention involving alterations in SL (stride length) based on body dimensions."

Another interesting finding from the Cavanagh and Williams study was that seven of the ten individuals studied employed strides that were longer than that predicted to be optimal. Of these, three overshot their optimal stride length by a considerable distance of 5 centimeters or more. Interestingly, in the study discussed earlier, Bryan Heiderscheit found that an increase in cadence of 5 percent from an individual runner's preferred value reduced stride length on average by about 5 centimeters. By combining the findings from these two studies (which is admittedly speculative), 30 percent of the runners from Cavanagh and Williams' study ran with a considerably longer than optimal stride length in terms of efficiency, and their strides were probably more impactful on their joints than if they ran at their optimal stride length. These would seem like obvious candidates for a bit of form work, and once again emphasizes why variation among individuals is always critical to take into account.

The authors conclude by stating the following: "The major implication of the results of this investigation is that well-trained runners are likely to run with a combination of SL (stride length) and SF (stride frequency) which is extremely close to their optimal condition," with the optimal condition being the one that requires the least expenditure of energy. The results of this study have left a lasting impression among coaches and running researchers, and it's not uncommon to hear experts claim that form change should not be pushed since runners automatically choose the optimal stride for their own body. There are a few problems with this viewpoint. First, most runners in Cavanagh and Williams' study chose a near optimal stride length, but not all—30 percent of them had stride lengths that were over 5 centimeters longer than optimal. Second, all of the subjects that Cavanagh and Williams studied were "well-trained" runners—all were running an average of 40 to 110 miles per week at the time the study was conducted. Thus, these were very experienced runners who'd had plenty of time to feel out their gait and converge on what might be their personal optimal stride. It's difficult to know if the same could be said for new-to-the-sport recreational runners who run ten to fifteen miles per week and are training for their first half-marathon. Cavanagh, one of the most thoughtful, conservative, and precise scientists to study running mechanics, points this out, saying "It would be of considerable interest to replicate this study with a group of beginning runners to determine if their deviations from the optimal conditions is greater than the group of well-trained or experienced runners used in this study."

Although not necessarily conducted on beginning runners, Dr. Joseph Hamill of the University of Massachusetts published a paper in 1995 in the journal *Human Movement Science* in which he and colleagues performed a similar analysis to Cavanagh and Williams on ten college students who were "physically active at the time of participation in the study but not necessarily training." They found that energy expenditure was actually lowest on average at a stride rate of plus 10 percent from preferred, though the results were not significantly different from economy at their preferred stride rate. These results call into question the suggestion that all runners automatically choose the stride that is most optimal for their own body, and suggest that there is a small window within which some amount of stride length optimization via form work could be of benefit. What's more, form work could benefit a runner both by improving his efficiency and by reducing the forces applied to the major joints of his legs.

One other possibility that Cavanagh mentions in his paper is the idea that his "subjects have adapted through training to the particular combinations of SL (stride length) and SF (stride frequency) which appear to be optimal for their current running styles. It may be that the optimal conditions for an individual can be changed by a period of prolonged training at a stride length which differed considerably from the optimal value." This is of possible relevance to the effects of footwear on form, especially since shoes can alter such things as stride length and stride frequency. What is still unknown is if or how we adapt over the long term to such changes. For example, if you start running barefoot, you might be quite inefficient at first with a new and unfamiliar combination of stride rate and stride length. However, as time passes and you get used to the new technique, you might find a new optimal combination, and your energy expenditure might end up lower than it was in shoes.

There is one study that puts into practice much of what we have been discussing by investigating if gait retraining can in fact make a runner more efficient. In a 1994 issue of the *Journal of Applied Physiology*, Don Morgan and colleagues published a study where they identified runners with non-optimal (i.e., inefficient) strides (about 20 percent of their sample of forty-five runners) and attempted to retrain their strides to make them more efficient. At the end of a three week training period, Morgan found that individuals with non-optimal strides who had received stride length training had shifted their freely chosen stride length toward their optimal stride length. Furthermore, energy expenditure at the new freely chosen stride length had decreased markedly—in other words, their new gait after the training period was more efficient than their old gait. Control individuals who did not receive training experienced no such changes.

This study shows that gait retraining does have the potential to shift running gait in positive ways, but they did not look at long term retention of the new gait. Do these people just revert to their old ways after the study is done? Although not geared toward investigating changes in efficiency, recent studies that have provided real-time feedback training to runners with a goal of reducing shock applied to the leg have shown that gait changes can be retained for extended periods after the training period has ceased, so the technique does have promise of lasting benefit. Additional studies like these are needed, and the answers that they provide will help all runners better understand the implications of efforts to modify their stride through form work or changes in footwear.

What About the Rest of the Body?

While much of this book has focused on the running body from the waist down, it's important to remember that what you do with the parts of the body from the waist up can also influence your running gait. In fact, form problems originating above the waist have the potential to influence both your efficiency and injury risk.

For example, research has suggested that deficiencies in hip flexor mobility can limit the ability of the hip to extend to help drive the body forward as you increase running speed. Your hip flexors (iliopsoas muscle) extend from your vertebrae, sacrum, and pelvis to an attachment on the thigh bone (femur). When the hip flexors contract, they swing the thigh forward and up as occurs when you are marching in place. How does one get tight hip flexors? One hypothesis is that sitting all day keeps the hip flexors in a shortened position, and this can ultimately lead to tightness and reduced mobility of these muscles.

So what do tight hip flexors have to do with running form above the waist? When you try to extend your thigh out behind the body during the late stance phase of the gait cycle (when the foot is preparing to leave the ground), the hip flexors stretch and become taut, thus limiting this extension. Excessively tight hip flexors can magnify this limitation. To compensate for limited extension at the hip joint and still allow the thigh to function to drive the body forward, you tend to instead tilt your pelvis forward, and this can in turn lead to excessive arching of the lower back. The combination of forward tilting of the pelvis and arching of the lower back has been suggested to be linked to both hamstring strains and lower back pain. So, while sitting in an office chair all day may not seem stressful to the body, it might just contribute to a chain of events leading to pain when you run.

In an article published on the *UVA Endurosport* blog, Jay Dicharry further discusses the influence of posture on running form. Dicharry sees many injured runners who exhibit poor posture when they run. In particular, he emphasizes that many runners tend to arch their lower back. Aside from potential direct effects this might have on the back itself, arching the lower back when you run has the effect of moving the center of mass backward, which in turn can cause the foot to land further in front of the center of mass. The end result is a longer stride. Dicharry suggests that maintaining a more neutral lower back position can help keep the stride shorter and reduce impact. How does one accomplish this? Aside from building a strong core and maintaining limber hip flexors, Dicharry suggests the simple cue to "Run tall!" With a bit of practice, improved posture can go a long way toward helping you iron out kinks in your form.

The arms also play an important role in your running. The primary role of arm swing is to help counterbalance trunk rotation caused by the alternating swing of the legs. Steve Magness, assistant coach to Alberto Salazar at the Nike Oregon Project, describes proper arm swing on his *Science of Running* blog:

> *The arm swing occurs from the shoulders, so that the shoulders do not turn or sway. It is a simple pendulum like forward and backward motion without shoulder sway or the crossing of the arms in front of your body. On the forward upswing the arm angle should decrease slightly with the hands in a relaxed fist. On the backswing they should swing back to just above and behind your hip joint for most running speeds. As running speed increases, the arm will swing back more, eventually culminating in going back and upwards in sprinting.*

Magness also feels that form problems manifested by the legs can sometimes be linked to problems with arm swing, writing that:

A lot of times we see something happening with the leg that is incorrect and immediately work on fixing the problem by adjusting how that particular leg is working. For example, if an athlete extends out with the lower leg, we immediately try and correct them by having them put their foot down sooner. Instead, the problem seen with the leg could simply be the symptom. The real cause could be in the arm swing. A delayed arm swing or one with a hitch in it causes a delay or hitch in the opposite lower leg. If you watch someone run, the arms and legs are timed up so they work perfectly in synch. If the runner has a problem with their arm swing that causes a delay in the typical forward and backward motion, such as turning it inwards or shoulder rotation, then the opposite leg must compensate for this delay. In many cases, the opposite leg extends outwards as a form of compensation. Therefore, it is important to look at the whole body and understand that the arms and legs are synched together and interact so that a problem in one of them, might simply be a way of compensation.

When Dicharry was asked if he ever looks to the arms for clues when examining an injured runner in his gait clinic, he mentioned that watching movement of the arms can provide "hints" regarding the source of problems that appear in the lower body. For example, he says that "a wide arm swing tells you that there is some type of lateral instability in the lower body, and an arm swing that crosses midline tells you that there is a rotational instability somewhere in the body. You combine that with information you get from doing screening tests and it can help you to track down things like chronic muscle imbalances."

The lesson here is an easy one to follow: runners tend to spend a disproportionate amount of time worrying about their legs and feet; but lifting their gaze a bit to the upper body can be revealing, and might just help them to identify, and possibly correct, the source of a chronic ache or pain in their lower limbs.

Conclusion

Overstriding has been recognized as a gait flaw for over a century. Science has now provided much-needed backup for the beliefs of running pioneers like Alfred Shrubb and Arthur Newton—excessively long strides decrease a runner's efficiency by increasing both braking forces and vertical movement of the center of mass, and increase potentially damaging forces applied to the joints.

Although most experienced runners tend to find a stride that mini-mizes energetic cost, some 20 to 30 percent of experienced runners may not be running at their optimal combination of stride rate and length. To put this in perspective, of the nearly 24,000 runners who completed the 2011 Boston marathon, some 5,000 or more might have been running with a less than optimal stride. The situation for less experienced runners is not as well understood, though some evidence suggests that increasing step rate by 10 percent (and thus reducing stride length) could improve efficiency by a small amount (or at least not incur any metabolic penalty), and also significantly reduce joint loading.

All of this suggests that many runners could benefit by including some amount of stride-shortening form work into their training arsenal. The emerging science on running form change suggests that positive ben-efits can be accrued via gait retraining (for example, improved efficiency, reduced shock), and that stride changes obtained through gait retraining can be retained as a new normal. Incorporating a bit of barefoot train-ing is one potentially useful approach as barefoot running tends to both shorten strides and reduce impact relative to running in shoes. Incorpo-rating speed work can also be helpful. If you are particularly concerned that an overstriding gait is causing you trouble, attempting a wholesale transition to a more barefoot-style form in your everyday running foot-wear may be well-worth considering.

If you decide to make an attempt at fine-tuning your gait, it's impor-tant to remember that tinkering with a form element like stride length involves some amount of risk—you don't want to create a new injury, and it's better to do nothing than to do harm. John Jerome, in his 1980 book *The Sweet Spot in Time*, provides some great insight from Peter Ca-vanagh on this topic. "If you change stride length, you change the action of almost every muscle in the body. A tiny little insignificant, innocent-looking change is really powerful as far as what its consequences are in the muscles of the body." We are learning how to harness this power, but as yet our understanding is imperfect, and caution is warranted.

In the final analysis, when it comes to form change, many unanswered questions still remain. For now, the wisest and most prudent course of action is to experiment individually, but avoid change for change's sake. Always remember that any experimentation should be conducted care-fully and gradually, and with clear understanding of the relative risks and rewards involved.

❦

CHAPTER 9

⟨⟨✕⟩⟩

Turning the Clock Back on Nutrition

The night before the race, we treated ourselves to a nice restaurant complete with a four-course meal of shrimp cocktail, baked potato, red wine, and ice cream.

—GRETE WAITZ, ON THE NIGHT BEFORE HER
FIRST NEW YORK CITY MARATHON WIN IN 1978

Diet is an overlooked aspect of achieving good running form. And by diet, we don't just mean trying to lose those extra pounds stubbornly clinging to the belly, thigh, or hips. Nutrition also concerns a lot more than being calorie-conscious, or knowing when to pop that energy gel into your mouth after an hour or two of running. Gait and eating well are intricately linked; a faulty diet can even lead to running injuries such as chronic knee pain, illiotibial band syndrome, and shin splints. It wasn't always this way.

Just as man was born to run, he was born to eat—only the right combination of real foods as they existed in nature. Right up to the time of the agricultural revolution about 10,000 years ago, the human diet was made up almost exclusively of vegetables, fruits, meat, fish, tubers, nuts and seeds. These basic staples provided the proper amount of protein for the repair of muscle, tissue, and organs; carbohydrates for prompt energy;

and fat for a healthy immune system and long-term energy. There was the occasional honey, but no processed sugar or vegetable oils, and an absence of all grains.

Because early man was an omnivore, he often needed to travel far and wide to satiate his hunger. He would regularly search out new foraging and hunting locations, just like modern-day restaurant diners do in San Francisco or Los Angeles. To fill their bellies, or at least keep from starving, our ancestral forebears were physically active as they looked for sustenance, and the food obtained was a reward for the energy and effort expended. In his book *Catching Fire: How Cooking Made Us Human*, Harvard anthropologist Richard Wrangham writes about chimpanzees in Ngogo, Uganda, which spend on average only a few minutes per day hunting for food, whereas men from modern hunter-gatherer societies hunt for between 1.8 and 8.2 hours per day. Women in modern hunter-gatherer societies are equally active. For example, Wrangham reports that among the Hadza tribe of Africa, women leave camp early in the morning to dig for tubers, and after several hours of work typically lug home at least 33 pounds of ekwa root (sometimes while carrying an infant). The women spend the rest of the day in camp cooking the collected food while waiting for the men to return from their hunt—the hope is that they will bring back meat to round out the evening meal. It's a hard life and the near-constant search for food is a central component.

The human diet witnessed a radical change when about sixty or seventy thousand years ago, the Stone Age set migrated from the African savanna and began its exodus to more northern regions in the Middle East and Near Asia. New research suggests this movement by foot may have occurred much earlier, triggered in part by global warming. By about 10,000 years ago, instead of hunting and foraging, the planting of seasonal crops such as barley and wheat took hold in this new environment, along with the raising of pigs, goats, chickens, and sheep. These farming and livestock developments supported the growth of villages and division of labor, but they also served to act as a necessary hedge against famine. Grains were harvested and stockpiled for hard times. And this is where gastronomic trouble began to affect humans, asking the body to revamp a digestive tract that had evolved for several million years in order to accommodate a very different type of diet.

"Humans, as a species, have been around for approximately 10,000 generations, and the human genus has been around for more than 100,000 generations. For all but the last 600 generations, our ancestors were hunter-gatherers," Harvard's Daniel Lieberman wrote in an 2011 op-ed piece for the *New York Times*. "Accordingly, the bodies we inherited are still mostly adapted to a hunter-gatherer way of life, which includes plentiful exercise, and a diet rich in protein and fiber, but low in saturated fat and simple sugars. Today's well-fed children may grow taller than a typical hunter-gatherer, and they have a much lower chance of dying young. But as standards of living rise throughout the world, so do obesity rates and related illnesses that are virtually unknown among hunter-gatherers such as adult-onset diabetes, coronary heart disease and cancer."

There's a growing belief in the scientific community that humans would be better off eating like they did during the Paleolithic period—instead of having three daily meals, they would nibble (yes, snacking!) throughout the day on vegetables, fruits, and nuts; and maybe there would be meat to be shared around the campfire (not unlike the family backyard barbecue). Paleolithic fruits, albeit not as sweet as today's varieties, included apples, dates, figs, plums, berries, and pears. Early man also noshed on edible plants such as ferns and cattails, though it'd be hard to find these items stocked in the produce section at say, Whole Foods.

This turning-back-the-clock approach to nutrition has generated many adherents, finding its way onto a plethora of blogs and bestseller lists with catchy book titles such as *The Stone Age Diet*, *The Caveman Diet*, *The Paleo Diet*, *The Hunter-Gatherer Diet*, *The Origin Diet*, and *The Evolution Diet*. For many followers of an early hominid diet, it's not a question of simply eating organic foods, non-farmed fish, free-range chicken, or grass-fed beef. Several other critical factors come into play. Like avoiding sugary treats and food made from processed grain.

"Our over-reliance on grain-based nutrition is especially problematic," says exercise physiologist Loren Cordain, PhD, author of *The Paleo Diet* and coauthor of *The Paleo Diet for Athletes*, and who is often considered to be the father or proverbial spear-carrier of the born-to-eat movement. Wheat intolerance and celiac disease, also known as gluten-sensitive enteropathy (gluten is a protein composite found in wheat and related species), are ticking time-bombs for chronic health woes, showing up as intestinal discomfort, allergies, liver problems, and depression. Wheat allergy can also affect the immune system, triggering low energy and chronic fatigue, two misdiagnosed symptoms found in endurance athletes who might be overindulging with their carb intake. And it's not only wheat that's problematic; other gluten-containing grains include durum, semolina, spelt, kamut, rye, and barley.

While there are close to 3,000 edible plants that have at one time been used as food, there are now only about twenty main crops that are cultivated throughout the world. Most of these crops, such as corn, have been so modified that their nutritional value is minimal at best. It's difficult to imagine how people would react if supermarkets were one day emptied of all rice, corn, and soy-based products.

In the past fifty or so years, as humans have become even less physically active, they have also become more dependent on sweets and highly processed food. All of those tasty snacks filled with starch, sugar, and cooked-in-artificial fat might please the palate, but this runaway addiction to junk food has contributed to a steady increase in obesity, hypertension, diabetes, and heart disease. In fact, obesity-related diseases account for nearly 10 percent of U.S. medical spending, or an estimated $147 billion a year. Each year, the average American consumes 140 pounds of high-fructose sweeteners in products such as fruit juice, soft drinks, breakfast cereals, and even tomato sauce. Americans now eat an average of 33 pounds of cheese a year—that is three times the 1970 amount; in fact, cheese has become the largest source of saturated fat in the nation's diet. According to a report issued in 2011 by the Trust for America's Health, the number of obese U.S. adults rose in sixteen states from the previous year, helping to push obesity rates in a dozen states above 30 percent.

So which single food item is the biggest culprit leading to a nation of supersized citizens? It's the potato, according to a recent study, "Changes in Diet and Lifestyle and Long-Term Weight Gain in Women and Men," which was published in the June 2011 issue of the *New England Journal of Medicine*. But it's not the potato in its natural form—you first need to slice *Solanum tuberosum*, cook it in oil and turn the pieces into chips or french fries. In the study, led by Dariush Mozaffarian, associate professor in the Harvard School of Public Health, long-term diet and lifestyle habits of more than 100,000 health professionals were analyzed. None of the subjects were obese at the start. Their weight was measured every four years for two decades. The average weight gain was seventeen pounds over the twenty-year period. The study found that a "daily serving {of the potato} containing 1 ounce (about 15 chips and 160 calories) led to a 1.69-pound uptick over four years. That's compared to sweets and desserts, which added 0.41 pound." Soda only added a pound each four year-period.

"There is no magic bullet for weight control," said a member of the research team, Dr. Frank Hu. "Diet and exercise are important for preventing weight gain, but diet clearly plays a bigger role."

The published study furthermore concluded: "Since weight stability requires a balance between calories consumed and calories expended, the advice to 'eat less and exercise more' would seem to be straightforward. However, weight gain often occurs gradually over decades (about 1 lb per year), making it difficult for most people to perceive the specific causes."

This might explain why weight gain and dieting remains such a maddening obsession among so many of us, including runners. But why as a society are we eating so poorly? Why have refined carbohydrates, sugar-fortified foods, artificial ingredients, packaged goods, and fast-food fare come to dominate the gustatory landscape? What are the other major health risks? These are all questions that have been discussed, analyzed, and dissected just about everywhere in the media, ranging from talk shows to weight-loss seminars to fitness magazines. Yet the bitter, unavoidable truth is that not much has changed. Every year, publishers come out with diet books promoting new weight-loss eating plans that were developed by a medical or health "expert", who is often a Hollywood celebrity or personal trainer to the stars. Many of these "breakthrough" titles have a knack of inching their way up the *New York Times* bestseller how-to list. Or some "nutritionist" will claim that a South American or African miracle fruit has special weight-loss and anti-oxidant properties.

But why should runners, who are fairly active individuals, be concerned about their diet? With all those calories being burned on a regular basis, aren't runners granted a nutritional exemption, a free lunch so to speak, when it comes to the ceaseless pleasures of food?

Hunter-Gatherer Fitness

An article about fitness and the hunter-gatherer lifestyle appeared in the *American Journal of Medicine* in 2010. The paper, which was written by James O'Keefe, MD, of the Mid America Heart Institute, in Kansas City, and three coauthors, including Loren Cordain, begins with the following overview: "Quantum improvements in technology such as those that spawned the agricultural revolution (350 generations ago), the industrial revolution (seven generations ago), and the digital age (three generations ago) have engendered large systematic reductions in the amount of physical work required by humans. Nonetheless, our innate exercise capabilities and requirements that evolved via natural selection over thousands of millennia remain essentially the same as for our Stone Age ancestors. Marked deviation from those indigenous exercise patterns predictably results in physical disability and disease."

So just how did Early Man spend the majority of his waking hours? Always on the move, hunting and foraging? Echoing Richard Wrangham's observation regarding daily activity among modern hunter-gatherers, the authors state that "except for the very young or the very old, everyone did a wide range of manual labors on a daily basis. Their activities of daily life were all the "exercise" that Stone Age people would have ever needed to maintain superb general fitness." But there's something more, a basic principle regarding rest and recovery that all overtrained runners should wisely heed. "Our ancient ancestors evolved an instinct compelling them to 'Move when you have to, and rest when you can.'"

They further explain the hard/easy lifestyle of hunter-gathers. Going all out every day on a hunt would have been far too impractical, not unlike asking an elite long-distance runner to train without ever taking rest days. "Hunter-gatherers would have likely alternated difficult days with less demanding days when possible. Their routines called for endeavors that promoted aerobic endurance, flexibility, and strength; thereby bestowing them with multi-faceted fitness that would have also conferred resiliency and reduced the likelihood of injury."

The authors cite estimates of average daily distances covered by Early Man. These numbers were in the range of six to sixteen kilometers. Carrying twenty kilograms of meat back to camp would have burned about 700 calories per hour for a 176-pound man. As for the typical daily energy expenditure associated with general physical activity, it would have been between 800 to 1200 calories—which is three to five times greater than the typical adult American today.

Judging strictly from a performance and lifestyle perspective, a runner who follows a healthy diet will have these advantages: be less prone to injury; have more stamina to train and race more efficiently; and a stronger immune system (which often means getting fewer colds). While a surprising number of elite runners have relatively poor diets, their great genes and metabolism often trump bad eating habits. Throughout his stellar reign in the 1970s, the nutritionally challenged Bill Rodgers was unstoppable and practically unbeatable, winning the Boston Marathon and New York City Marathons four times each. The Boston Beanpole never gained weight despite a crazy diet—he'd eat cold pizza topped with mayonnaise for breakfast. He also had a fondness for Fritos and packaged macaroni and cheese. During his prime, Alan Webb, who's the current U.S. record-holder in the mile, followed a diet taken right out of an *Animal House* cookbook, living off Ramen noodles, fried chicken wings, greasy Chinese food, and McDonald's.

Anton Krupicka, a two-time winner of the Leadville 100 ultra, is a popular, almost mythic, figure in mountain-running circles. With his unkempt beard and long hair, combined with a preference for running topless in just shorts and minimalist shoes, the Boulder, Colorado resident, who lives several months at a time in his camper pickup nicknamed The Roost, looks like he's been quantum-teleported from the Paleo era. Photos of him show nary a surplus of excess body fat. Considering the heavy mileage Krupicka regularly logs—fifteen to thirty-five miles barefoot out of a total of up to 180 weekly miles—it's also critical that he must eat a lot to fuel his body.

Krupicka wrote about his diet on his blog: "I consciously try to eat a lot of fresh, local fruits and vegetables, often purchased from the local farmer's market (April to November), but I definitely tend to eat a whole lot of straight-up carbs/sugar in the forms of pasta, breads, muffins, scones, cookies, Nutella on tortillas, chai, etc. I probably eat too much sugar. I don't eat any fast food, except for Illegal Pete's (local Chipotle-style burritos) here in Boulder, if that qualifies.

"In terms of eating enough to handle the mileage, I don't have a secret diet, however, I think I probably do have a fairly unique (i.e. slow) metabolism, because I don't feel like I eat a ridiculous amount. Or, maybe the quantity I eat is all I've ever known and it actually is a ridiculous amount. Or, maybe other people just eat too much relative to the amount of activity they have in their lives thereby making my diet not feel so out of place. I don't know."

During long training runs and racing, Krupicka regularly depends on GU for energy replenishment, popping a carb-rich gel into his mouth every twenty minutes along with sips of water. He writes: "During training, on runs of four hours of more I generally eat one GU per hour after the first two hours. I have found this to usually be enough but certainly not ideal in terms of energy needs. In the summer I will carry a 20 oz. bottle on runs over two hours (and refill at streams when I feel the need). The plan is to never deprive myself of calories, and hopefully the restricted use in training has increased my body's ability to metabolize fat and hold onto water and salt."

It should be noted that the specific combination of ingredients contained in an energy gel like GU isn't found in natural foods in their raw state: natural fructose (fruit sugar), complex carbs in the form of maltodextrin, citrates (potassium citrate, sodium citrate and citric acid), and branched chain amino acids such as leucine, valine and isoleucine, histidine, which is another essential amino acid, and antioxidant vitamins C and E, and some sea salt. Energy gels are popular because they give a quick blast of carbohydrates that helps fuel a hard-working body, and more importantly, they are easy to consume on the run. However, some endurance runners have found that opting for whole foods as fuel on the run can be a more enjoyable, and perhaps healthier option when time is not the primary concern.

In *Born to Run*, Christopher McDougall wrote that the diet of the ultrarunning Tarahumara Indians of Mexico was based on dense, natural, energy-rich foods such as pinole, which is a coarse flour made from ground-roasted maize (corn) kernels, and chia, a seed rich in protein, fiber, and omega-3 fatty acids. (Chia was an important crop for ancient Aztecs.) These seventeen words McDougall included in one passage—"a tablespoon of chia is like a smoothie made from salmon, spinach, and human growth hormone"—likely accounted for a sudden spike in chia-seed sales in health food stores in the U.S.

Many *Born to Run* readers were also introduced to ultrarunning phenom Scott Jurek, who has long been a dominant force on the ultra circuit. McDougall described the seven-time winner of Western States 100 as "a pure racing animal. The top ultrarunner in the country, maybe in the world, arguably of all time." Unlike the Tarahumara who do eat meat—it's just not readily available—Jurek is a vegan, and has been one for years. In a 2010 interview with *New York Times* food writer Mark Bittman, Jurek talked about his diet growing up, saying it was "very Midwest—meat and potatoes." In college, he began to eat better, beause he "saw how much disease is lifestyle related," and thus he began charting his nutritional journey towards only "real food, eating the way people have been eating for thousands of years."

He started eating less meat and more fish; then dairy went. Soon, his diet became all vegetarian. "It's really a mental barrier," he told the *Times* reporter, "and I get that all {my calories} from plant sources. It's not hard, either. I like to eat, and I don't have to worry about weight management. All I need is a high-carbohydrate diet with enough protein and fat."

And just how many calories does he require each day to support an ultraunner's lifestyle? Jurek said that he needs to consume between 5,000 and 8,000 calories per day. As for specific foods, Bittman writes:

> *He focuses on three main meals. Breakfast is key: it might be a 1,000-calorie smoothie, with oil, almonds, bananas, blueberries, salt, vanilla, dried coconut, a few dates and maybe brown rice protein powder. Unless he is doing a long run, which for him is seven hours, or about 50 miles, he eats after his first workout. Lunch and dinner are huge salads, whole grains, potatoes and sweet potatoes, and usually beans of some sort or a tempeh-tofu combination.*

Nor does Jurek feel the least bit apologetic about being a vegan. "None of this is weird. If you go back 300 or 400 years, meat was reserved for special occasions, and those people were working hard. Remember, almost every long-distance runner turns into a vegan while they're racing, anyway—you can't digest fat or protein very well."

In another interview with the *Huffington Post,* Jurek discussed how he enjoys eating whole foods during both races and on training runs:

> *People are always surprised when they see me during a race eating a burrito or a falafel wrap. But when I'm out for six, seven hours, I love to sit on a mountain pass and just enjoy a good hummus wrap or a bean-and-rice burrito. Real food like that. I just pop it out of my waist pack." Jurek believes that his diet has played a big role in his success as a runner, saying that his decision to become a vegan "was one of those things that really impacted my health and recovery and training, and it's been a big reason for why I've been so consistent with races and pumping out serious results. A lot of people think*

ultramarathoning has long-term damaging effects on your body. That's where I feel like the diet has played a huge role. As a result of it, my body is able to withstand all the demands I put on it. It's longevity in the sport.

Weighty Matters

Many runners think little about the short-term and long-term effects of their reliance on high-fructose sports drinks, sugar-fortified energy bars, and all-you-can-eat pre-race pasta banquets where participants feel entitled to gorge themselves like kings and queens. And while these runners often overlook critical aspects of a poor diet, or wonder why they are still overweight given all the mileage they log, they seemed to be more concerned by how many ounces their running shoes weigh.

This obsession is actually supported by science. Research has shown that reducing shoe weight can result in a modest improvement to a runner's efficiency. In his book *Lore of Running*, the world-famous South African exercise physiologist Timothy Noakes writes about how an average a runner will see an approximately one percent reduction in the oxygen cost of running (an estimator of energy expenditure or economy) per 3.5 oz reduction in shoe weight. So if a 3:30 marathoner goes from wearing 11.5-ounce training shoes to 8-ounce flats for his next race, that could theoretically translate into an overall savings of 126 seconds, or just over two minutes (a savings of almost five seconds per mile).

But try looking at this same scenario from another angle—body weight. What if this lighter-shod runner is say, ten pounds overweight? Tom Osler, a top ultrarunner in the 1960s who later became a math professor and author of *The Serious Runner*, conducted a comprehensive study of runners and found that for every extra pound one carries, that person will be 2.5 seconds per mile slower. If a marathoner is carting ten extra pounds, he will be going 25 seconds slower per mile; it will take him an extra eleven minutes to finish the marathon! (And thus negating the two minutes he saved by wearing lighter shoes.) Even more importantly, his heart, lungs, and muscles will have been working harder since he has more body mass.

In a 2007 paper in the *Journal of Experimental Biology*, a team of researchers from the University of Colorado dug deeper into the relationship between body weight and running economy by either strapping lead weights to the waist of runners, or reducing their effective weight by suspending them from a harness while running on a treadmill. They found that the effort required to support body weight comprises 74 percent of the metabolic cost of running, and reported that "a 10 percent increase in body mass increased metabolic rate by 14 percent." They suggest that this added cost could be explained by "greater muscle activation to stabilize these loads (either trunk and/or leg musculature), recruitment of less economical motor units (motor units are groups of fibers in muscles) or an impaired ability to re-utilize elastic energy."

Body Mass Index

The Body Mass Index, or BMI, has long been considered the standard for measuring the amount of fat in a person's body. The Body Mass Index is defined as the individual's body weight (in kilograms) divided by height in meters squared. For example, if you are five-ten and 185 pounds, your BMI is approximately 26.5. Generally, a BMI of 25 or above indicates a person is overweight; 30 or above indicates obesity. A person with a higher BMI is considered to be at greater risk for heart disease, diabetes, and other weight-related problems.

BMI Categories:
Underweight = <18.5
Normal weight = 18.5–24.9
Overweight = 25–29.9
Obesity = BMI of 30 or greater

The BMI was created in the mid-1800s by the Belgian social scientist Adolphe Quetelet, who was investigating "social physics," or methods of comparing different populations. But according to new research, the BMI may not be as accurate as originally conceived. A research group from Michigan State University and Saginaw Valley State University measured the BMI of more than four hundred college students—some of whom were athletes and some not—and found that in most cases the students' BMI did not accurately reflect their percentage of body fat. While BMI can be calculated quickly and without expensive lab equipment, BMI categories fail to take into account factors such as frame size and muscle mass. Also, BMI is often used as an imprecise substitute for percent body fat. "The overlying issue is the same criteria for BMI are used across the board," said Joshua Ode, a PhD student in the MSU Department of Kinesiology, who assisted in the study. "Many athletes have huge BMIs because of muscle mass, but in many cases are not fat."

The U.S. Army stopped using the BMI because of too many overweight recruits—27.1 percent of all eighteen-year-olds who applied to join the military in 2006 were overweight. So the Army changed its fat policy to make it more lenient. New recruits are now measured based upon a statistical table that lists an appropriate weight for any given height.

Some researchers think that waist size is a better indicator than BMI in determining one's overall health. *New York Times* health reporter Tara Parker-Pope wrote that "many studies of both men and women now suggest that it is not how much you weigh but where you carry your weight that matters most to your health."

In the March 2008 issue of the *Journal of Clinical Epidemiology*, a study showed that body mass index is the 'poorest' indicator of cardiovascular health, and that waist size is a much better way to determine, for both sexes, who is at a higher risk for hypertension, [type 2] diabetes and elevated cholesterol."

Is there an ideal body mass for a runner? The ideal weight and optimal fat-to-lean ratio varies considerably for men and women as well as by age. The average adult body fat is 15 to 18 percent for men and 22 to 25 percent for women. The minimum percent of body fat considered safe for good health is 5 percent for males and 12 percent for females. Runners tend to be at the low end due to their increased lean weight, or muscle mass. Elite marathoners can have as low as 3 percent body fat. When Frank Shorter (five feet, ten inches) won the Olympic gold medal in the marathon in 1972, he weighed just 135 pounds with an alarmingly low body fat of 2.2 percent.

There's another important consideration regarding a runner's extra body weight—it's what this additional burden can do to one's joints over a long distance or sustained period of time. The amount doesn't have to be much, maybe 5, 10 or 15 pounds, but it adds up in a sport so strongly characterized by repetitive impact. Each time a runner strikes the ground, the feet, shins, knees, and hips feel the force of the collision between body and ground. "The ground reaction forces when walking are 1.1 times body weight, and 2.2 to 2.7 times body weight when running," says Jay Dicharry. "More mass means more force—obviously!" The laws of physics would seem to suggest that extra body weight will amplify that ground-reaction force. So should heavier runners opt for shoes with more cushion, rigid support, and thicker heels, in order to lessen the foot-striking impact? Isn't this what these runners have been led to believe for years?

Well, the answer is "no," according to biomechanical expert Dr. Casey Kerrigan. "Being overweight increases the risk for knee osteoarthritis so most certainly for a heavy runner, consideration of the forces through the knee joint should be given the highest priority," she says. "I think a heavier Clydesdale-type runner should stay clear of any cushioned shoe from the start. Because, indeed, although the idea that a traditional running shoe increases forces through the knees is counterintuitive, that is exactly what we found in the gait laboratory. But the increased forces we found were not at impact. The peak forces that are associated with knee osteoarthritis always occur later in the stance phase when the foot is fully planted—in midstance. This is the case regardless of running form or whether or not someone is wearing shoes—minimal or otherwise. It is at this point in the gait cycle, when the foot is fully planted, and the foot and the lower leg are absorbing and releasing the body weight in preparation for the next step, that joint torques (which relate to joint forces), and really all stresses and strains related to common injuries, are the highest. This is the point when runners are at risk for osteoarthritis, and virtually ever other major injury, including stress fractures."

Kerrigan maintains that a cushioned shoe "does not increase joint torques at impact. But what cushioning does do, which is harmful, is make the joints work harder, later, in midstance. Despite all the so-called advances in foam, gel and air filled bladder technologies, the typical midsole compresses and releases out of sync with the rise and fall of the body weight. By working out of sync, a cushioned midsole makes the joints (and all injury prone areas for that matter) have to work harder, which we see by way of the greater joint torques."

In the final analysis, Kerrigan emphatically believes that "the heavy runner should run in a shoe with no cushioning."

Breakdown in Form

Still, it bears repeating: with all the training they do, why are many run-ners still carrying around extra pounds? And what does it mean in terms of performance? While many overweight people take up running to lose weight, and are often quite successful at shedding pounds as part of a healthy eating and lifestyle turnaround, if you go to any big city mara-thon, half-marathon, or 10K, a significant number of runners in the field are, to put it not quite diplomatically, clearly tipping the scales.

These overweight runners are at a disadvantage when it comes to maintaining optimal running form. Once again, the weight doesn't have to be all that much—a slight paunch can throw a gait out of bal-ance. Dr. Steve Gangemi, of Chapel Hill, North Carolina is a comple-mentary sports medicine specialist and a 16-time Ironman finisher. As a holistic practitioner skilled in manual muscle biofeedback, Gangemi doesn't wear shoes while treating patients, and has a popular website on injury prevention for endurance athletes called Sock Doc. He has a particular interest in gait and performance. "Let's face it, if you're a big person, you're going to be slower than someone smaller, provided your fitness levels are identical," he says. "But studies don't take into ac-count where the weight is and how it's actually affecting your body. For example, large thighs on a runner are most likely going to slow him or her down more than someone with big upper arms. Excess fat is going to slow one down more than more muscle; it's towing extra weight and not giving anything back in return. Excess weight in certain areas can definitely affect gait."

Many male recreational runners have a tendency to be soft around the middle. The belly bulge, says Gangemi, "is usually due to eating too many unhealthy, high-glycemic carbs that get stored as body fat. That excess weight on the front of the body is going to cause the body to compensate so the runner is more sway-back, which is an exaggerated forward curvature of the lower back. Sway-back occurs as the shoulders are thrown back to compensate for excessive weight on the abdomen, and puts more pressure on the lumbar spine. That, in turn, will put more stress on the back of the knees, hamstrings, calves, and create more of a heel-strike landing. So having a gut can result in symptoms that are ulti-mately diagnosed as plantar fasciitis, heel spurs, and tendonitis. Further compensations can develop after that. In this case, the extra stress on the calf muscles in the back of the lower leg (the gastrocnemius and soleus) will then result in more of a workload being distributed to the front of the lower leg (the tibialis anterior primarily) and next thing you know, shin splints appear."

Okay, so let's say you are an average-size 5'10", 180-pound male, who is ten pounds over the goal of achieving six-pack ab status. To see firsthand how these pounds—which is just over five percent of your total body weight—can affect your gait, grab a 10-pound weight or heavy rock, put it a front-carrying fanny pack, and go for a short run. Feel the difference in your stride, body positioning, and even foot strike! Imagine running with that extra weight for a 10K or half-marathon.

"You actually don't need much to change gait," adds Gangemi. "The gait is also going to be significantly affected by the type of body fuel a runner is burning, even more than by additional weight. Anaerobic running that is done at a high heart rate using primarily sugar, or glucose, for fuel will result in many more muscle imbalances long before the runner who is going aerobic, which is at a lower heart rate and burns more body fat for fuel. The muscles throughout the entire body have such a strong connection to body chemistry and changes in glucose metabolism that they will soon fatigue when their glycogen stores are used up as a result of overtraining and in racing. Then, the gait changes. The feet land differently—they kick out or land with a harder strike. The center of gravity shifts. The legs get heavier. Body weight, no matter fat or muscle, or whether in the hips, glutes, or belly now takes its toll on the tiring runner."

In fact, you often see an increase in deteriorating running form just after the midway portion of a marathon, as the slower runners tap out their glycogen stores, and it only gets worse the closer they get to the finish line, often stumbling forward like inebriated frat boys after last call.

Body Fat

Dr. Phil Maffetone is also a complementary sports medicine practitioner, former coach to world-champion triathletes and endurance runners, and author of several books, including most recently, *The Big Book of Health and Fitness*. Since the 1980s, he has been studying body fat and athletes. His theory of why many runners are overweight is interesting because it hits upon touchy, controversial themes. "The issue of body fat remains a sensitive one for runners," he says. "On one hand, many believe that with all the training they do, their body fat should melt right off. But the reality is something quite different: they don't see that happening; in fact, higher than expected body fat is common among runners. Diet plays an important role in burning off excess body fat, but it also requires steady aerobic training that will turn your body into a fat-burning machine."

Carbs can only get you so far in terms of energy and endurance. The body has enough stored glycogen for about three hours (your body doesn't need supplementary carbs in the form of gels, bars, or beverages in a 5K or 10K). Then the gas tank is empty and you begin to experience the dreaded bonk. But the body has an untapped store of available fat that can be utilized as energy. That is why you can go several weeks without eating, but it's not something we'd recommend even if you are a contestant on one of those weight-loss reality television shows.

"The problem of excess body fat often begins when runners are in their twenties and thirties," continues Maffetone. "This period marks a change in metabolism. The body no longer tolerates certain dietary imbalances, non-optimal training, and daily stress that one's golden youth once easily brushed aside. Once you reach your mid- to late-twenties, several physiological functions begin to diminish. These include maximum oxygen uptake, maximum heart rate, lung capacity, muscle mass, and strength. The rate of decline is dependent upon overall fitness and health, especially aerobic capacity. As these age-related changes take place, body fat content tends to rise. But for an aging runner, who is fit and healthy, these typical declines in body composition—more fat, less muscle—don't occur.

"Restricting calories as a means of losing body weight is the most common approach used in the weight-loss industry and by individuals, especially among runners. About 95 percent of those who go on a calorie-restricted diet will fail in the long run. Runners often count calories to reduce or avoid too much body fat. By restricting calories, runners risk not supplying sufficient energy for optimal training. Of those who lose weight initially with calorie restriction, most will gain it back—plus more—in the end. Moreover, most will not lose body fat. Much of this problem is due to the fact that by restricting calories, one's metabolism is adversely reduced, with the result of eventually storing more body fat."

Okay, we know that a weight-reducing diet before an important race is a recipe for disaster, but what are the typical barriers that stand in the way of having a whippet-thin runner's body like many top elites? Here's Maffetone's take: "The three most common obstacles in relation to reducing body fat to healthy levels are carbohydrate intolerance, excess stress, and lack of good nutrition as supplied by a healthy diet. As we get older, we also become more resistant to insulin, which causes us to be more carbohydrate intolerant. So, even if we eat the same amount of refined carbohydrates we could eat at a younger age without a problem, it now turns to fat. This is an oversimplification but a good example of how our body changes over time. Most importantly, a diet rich in highly processed, high-glycemic foods—wheat, corn, sugar, and potatoes—converts to belly fat all too easily."

And what is Maffetone's diet recommendation for runners? "Natural carbohydrates, fats, and proteins. In addition, water and fiber are vital as well as vitamins, minerals, and phytonutrients. Most are easily available from a healthy real-food diet, especially when about ten servings of vegetables and fruits are consumed each day. Also beware of so-called health food store items that are high in sugar and calories and are unhealthy. Organic junk food can make you fat fast."

Maffetone's nutritional advice seems a lot like the Paleo diet, which is a lot like the 40-30-30 diet, or the Mediterranean eating plan. In the end, it really doesn't matter what you call your diet, so long as it's healthy and balanced, and avoids processed fare, refined sugars, refined grains, manufactured vegetable oil, dairy (primarily a concern for only those who are lactose intolerant), and artificial flavoring and ingredients. For example, the modern 40–30–30 diet—40 percent carbs, 30 percent protein, 30 percent fats—is an attempt to replicate the pre-grain eating habits of early man.

We have all seen those clever Geico car insurance ads: "So easy a caveman could do it." When choosing your food, it should be the same, but it isn't. That's because how we think about nutrition mirrors social, cultural, and even athletic trends and popular opinion. "Ours is a culture where a meal is measured by how fast it's served or how many grams of fat it may contain," wrote Michael Pollan in a *New York Times* essay aptly titled, "The National Eating Disorder," which later became the basis for his first bestselling book, *The Omnivore's Dilemma*. "We ignore, to our detriment, the wonderful social aspects of a long leisurely lunch that one experiences in other parts of the world. We have become, in the midst of our astounding abundance, the world's most anxious eaters. How we eat, and even how we feel about eating, may in the end be just as important as what we eat. So we've learned to choose our foods by the numbers (calories, carbs, fats, R.D.A.s, price, whatever), relying more heavily on our reading and computational skills than upon our senses. Indeed, we've lost all confidence in our senses of taste and smell."

The heart-healthy Mediterranean diet, which is a good practical model of sensible eating, is largely based on vegetables and fruits. And this leads one straight to Pollan's advice about how to rehabilitate the Western diet, which has been overtaken by nutritionism, fast-food addiction, packaged and processed foods, questionable meat-industry practices, and gargantuan agri-business. Pollan emphatically states at the outset of *In Defense of Food*, "Eat food. Not too much. Mostly plants." By basing your diet on those seven words—an easy enough regimen to follow—he argues that healthy eating is within everyone's reach. It is neither complicated nor confusing. It's a lesson all runners should heed.

Improving upon a faulty diet can lead to noticeable results, even within the space of several weeks. You might find yourself with newfound energy on your training runs. Or your race times have started to drop. Perhaps that lingering cold is no longer lingering. Unlike the slow, gradual adaptation process that is absolutely essential if you happen to make slight changes to your running form, or decide to go with more minimalist footwear, the great thing about eating healthier foods is knowing that your body will start benefiting right away. There's no breaking-in period. There's no long, drawn-out transitional period. Maffetone even says, "All it takes is one good, healthy meal for your body to respond in a positive manner." Diet isn't a zero-sum game of calories-in versus calories-out. It's where those calories come from that makes the real difference.

⚬∞⚬

Conclusion

I once ran thirty-one miles and after that there was nothing in the world I thought I couldn't do.

—KATHRINE SWITZER

Humans evolved to be distance runners. But modern runners frequently get hurt, sometimes badly enough to force them to give up the activity that their bodies should be finely tuned to perform. This is both puzzling and unfortunate, and this book was an attempt to explore some of the potential reasons why injuries are so common among today's runners.

Where do we go from here? Is there a bulletproof way to run injury-free? We would be naïve to think that we could provide a decisive answer to that question in these pages. Many of the topics that we have discussed here are currently the subject of passionate and sometimes fiery debate, and the search for answers about the causes of running injuries is far from over. In fact, it's only just beginning. And it's not just runners themselves who are making their voices heard and interest felt. Footwear scientists, biomechanical experts, running coaches, podiatrists, physical therapists, specialty running stores, and footwear designers are taking an active role on this exciting new front—and with each contributing their own unique expertise. Collectively, this is a good thing for runners. Progress is being made, and we hope that this will lead to a significant draw down in the number of running injuries. We may not have all of the answers right now, but it's a bold and invigorating time to be a runner. By all accounts, the lively discussion about footwear and form will continue. New developments, findings, and insights will emerge.

To help the conversation move forward, allow us to summarize the key points from *Tread Lightly:*

1. **We evolved to run, but we typically don't run like our ancestors.** Convincing evidence exists to support the hypothesis that humans are a species uniquely adapted to running long distances at a relatively slow pace. Furthermore, running provides numerous positive health benefits. However, the modern runner is in many ways far removed from his or her running ancestry. Differences between ancestral and modern runners may predispose us to injuries that were uncommon in our more distant history.

2. **Runners will always get hurt.** Almost all running injuries result from repetitive stress, and runners are stubborn and quite good at overstressing their bodies. As long as we continue to overtrain and push ourselves to the limit in our workouts and races, we are bound to succumb to an injury at some point. Being smart in your training and respecting your limits are probably the two things most likely to reduce your risk of getting hurt.

3. **Runners can take measures to reduce their repetitive stress load.** Here are some valuable strategies:

    a. Don't do high-intensity workouts frequently unless you know your body can handle it.

    b. Include easy days and recovery runs in your training.

    c. Don't switch to a new shoe (minimalist or otherwise) or barefoot running and proceed immediately with normal training loads. This is particularly true if the shoe you are transitioning to is structurally different than your previous shoe in a significant way (for example, if there's a lower heel, different level of cushioning, or support). It's best to work a new shoe into your footwear rotation gradually so that your body can adapt to it. Also, if something feels wrong after several runs in a shoe, try something else and see if it gets better.

    d. Rotate among several shoes if you can afford multiple pairs, particularly if you run all of your miles on roads. Keeping a rotation that includes a long distance shoe, a trail shoe, and perhaps a racing flat or barefoot-style/minimalist shoe for form work and strengthening might be an approach worth trying. Mix it up a bit when it comes to footwear, but don't go overboard to the point where you never adapt to anything. Different shoes will stress your body in slightly different ways, and using a mix might help reduce repetitive stress.

e. If you don't already, do some running on trails. Trail running is a very different type of workout than road running, and a big part of the reason why is that you are typically running over uneven terrain. This helps to keep your legs working in different ways, breaks the repetitive stress cycle so typical of road running, and makes your legs overall stronger. Trails are also typically softer and more forgiving than asphalt and concrete, which can reduce the rate of force application (loading rate) even if impact force doesn't necessarily change on the softer surface.

f. Try to avoid running the same route, over the same distance, at the same pace, in the same shoes on every run. Again, mix things up—change speeds, run hills, and explore new routes. The more repetitive your workouts are, the more repetitive the stresses you experience are; consequently, the more likely it is that your body might break down.

g. Incorporate some amount of low-impact cross training. You can get a solid aerobic workout that will benefit your running by doing an activity like biking, swimming, a gym workout, or even a long walk or hike. Because these activities are low impact, they allow you to get in a workout that will benefit your physiology without further damaging your anatomy.

h. Above all else, take time to rest when you feel you need it. Your body is good at telling you something is wrong, so don't let a slight ache turn into a major problem. You're far better off taking a few days off than risking a severe injury and being sidelined for a month or more.

4. **Shoes are not evil.** Yes, our ancestors evolved to run barefoot. However, the vast majority of modern runners (co-authors included) are going to wear shoes most of the time. It's likely true that shoes of any type, even the most minimal, change how one runs, and the influence of these changes on running injury risk is a topic of active and intense scientific research. It's important to recognize shoe-induced changes in one's running, understand their implications (positive or negative),

and continue to study whether one might benefit by attempting to adopt a more barefoot-style stride while running in shoes.

5. **On finding the "perfect" shoe.** There is not a single perfect shoe for all runners. Each of us is different due to our genetics, physical makeup, training background, past history of shoe use, and so on. As a result, the shoe that works for one person may not work for you. The challenge is to find the shoe that works best for your individual body. Some people will be able to tolerate a wide range of footwear types, whereas others might have more specific needs. Science is still struggling to find good answers as to what any individual should wear or not wear on their feet, and the best advice supported by the scientific literature is to wear shoes that are comfortable. Comfort may be important, but finding the right shoes should be based on how they feel on the run, not how they feel while standing in a store. Shop at stores that let you take shoes for a test run—a shoe that seems ideal while standing in them might feel awful on the run, and a shoe that feels "off" while standing might feel great when you are moving. Above all else, don't be afraid to experiment—you may have to run in several different types of shoe before you find what works best for you. The only "perfect" running shoe is the one that helps to keep you off the couch.

6. **Be careful in shoe stores.** Runners should take much of what they are told in many shoe stores with a dose of healthy skepticism. Don't feel compelled to buy insoles. Be wary of a salesperson who gives you a selection of shoes based on your sitting or standing arch height. Don't put too much stock in prescriptions based on degree of pronation observed on a treadmill (and even less on pronation observed when you walk across a store carpet). The pronation control model may be useful at the extremes or as a starting point for looking at shoes, but runners shouldn't feel locked in for life if told that they "overpronate." Overpronation "diagnoses" are typically highly subjective and will likely vary depending on who is looking at you—go to three stores, and you may be told three different things. What's more, there isn't strong evidence that overpronation is a huge risk factor for injury. In stores, look for knowledgeable, open-minded sales clerks—people with broad experience with lots of shoes who are not tied to any particular dogma. Tell them what you like in a shoe—firm or soft, wide

or narrow, high heel or low heel, arch support or flat insole—they can narrow down choices for you based on far more than just pronation control.

7. **Avoid change for change's sake.** Don't feel compelled to switch shoes if what you are using is working well. If motion-control shoes keep you out on the road, then stick with them! If ultra-minimal shoes meet your needs, great! If barefoot feels best, go with it! The most important thing for a runner is simply to keep running—for personal enjoyment, exercise, competition, losing weight, reducing stress, and so on.

8. **Consider your choice of casual, everyday shoes.** If you spend a great deal of your waking hours in some kind of shoe, then the shoe you choose to wear for most of the day likely has greater long-term impact on your feet than what you wear on a half-hour or hour run. Find shoes that respect the shape of your feet and that don't constrict your toes. *You have a foot size, not shoe size.* If possible, wear flat shoes with low or no heels that don't contribute to potential shortening of your calf muscles and Achilles tendons, particularly if you tend toward running in shoes with a low heel. Fashion will likely always trump sensibility for many people, but if you truly value your foot health, then avoid ill-fitting shoes.

9. **Keep your children active, and allow their feet and form to develop naturally.** A child's footwear could heavily influence his or her long-term foot health as an adult. Similarly, our adult running form could have its roots in motor patterns we develop in childhood. Children need to be physically active, they should spend lots of time barefoot, and when wearing shoes, they should be provided footwear that allows their feet and gait to develop as freely and as naturally as possible. It is the role of parents to choose sensible shoes for their children.

10. **There is no such thing as "perfect" running form.** There is only a "best" running form for each individual given the situation in which he or she is running and the peculiarities of his or her own anatomy, physiology, and personal history. Unfortunately, many runners have poor, or less than optimal form, and this could possibly be the fault of their shoes. If you watch slow motion video of recreational runners you will quickly realize just how common overstriding and heel-mashing are. We're not talking about all forms of heel striking here, but rather the

extended leg, nearly locked knee, toes pointing to the sky at contact kind of gait. A runner can heel strike and do just fine—we truly believe this. But, the massive overstrider may be at risk, and overbuilt modern shoes seem to make the overstride much more likely to occur.

11. **On changing running form.** The most important question is whether an individual should even make an attempt to alter his or her running form. Perhaps the safest answer is that if you are running well and getting what you want from the sport, then you don't mess with success. Attempting to change your form could create problems where they previously did not exist. However, some individuals (perhaps a significant percentage) do not run with a form that allows for optimal efficiency, and some might be running with a form that can lead to an increased risk of injury.

How do you know if you might have a form problem? The first tipoff would be a chronic injury that continually recurs. It might be due to your form, or it might not; but getting some help is encouraged. You can start by simply filming yourself on a treadmill or having someone film you out on the road. Look for things like an overstriding gait (does your foot land well in front of your knee?) or excessive joint motion. If you are genuinely concerned, see a professional—there are lots of health care practitioners (physical therapists, podiatrists, chiropractors) with expertise in analyzing running gaits, so ask around and try to find one in your area. They can dissect your gait critically and identify problem areas. They can also offer suggestions and provide exercises that might help you improve your stride.

Because many runners will attempt to alter their gait on their own, here are some recommendations:

a. **Be careful, and make changes gradually!** Make sure that any attempted form change does not do harm, and respect the fact that altering your stride is going to stress your body in ways that it is likely not accustomed to. Take a gradual approach and allow your body to adapt slowly.

b. **Don't force foot-strike changes.** Many runners equate "form change" solely with a change in foot strike. Because one tends to land on the forefoot when one runs barefoot, it's tempting to suggest that this is the way *all* humans were meant to run. The problem with this line of thinking is that some individuals will hear or read about this and then go out and try to force a forefoot landing. This can result in an exaggerated attempt at a forefoot strike, with the runner almost tiptoeing down the road (often combined with an overstride). Running like this can put immense stress on the feet and lower legs, and could be downright dangerous. Avoid a single-minded focus on foot strike if you attempt to alter your running form.

c. **Consider stride rate and stride length.** Preventing an overstride may be more important and more practical than messing with the specifics of which part of your foot first contacts the ground. So, rather than focusing on foot strike, consider instead an attempt at a modest increase in step rate (say 5 to 10 percent from your baseline cadence) or a decrease in stride length. To reduce stride length, consider using cues to "land close to your body," "put your foot down behind you," or Bill Bowerman's cue to "land after your foot has started to swing back." Try visualizing landing with a vertical shin. Even a tactic as simple as trying to make less noise when you run can work—different people will succeed with different cues, so find the one that works best for you. What you may find is that by simply working on your stride length, your foot strike adapts on its own.

d. **Add some speed work.** Running fast can help you to fine-tune your form. Hit the track with a pair of flats and incorporate some intervals or repeats into your training repertoire. Go easy at first since speed increases injury risk, but you may find that running fast in less shoe allows you to feel out your stride in a way that is hard to do in cushioned trainers on easy runs.

e. **Try running barefoot.** Even if you have no intention of becoming a full-time barefoot runner, incorporating some barefoot running into your training is a great way to work on your form. Removing the interference between your feet and the ground will allow you to feel out your gait better, and will force you to adapt to a shorter, less impactful stride. You can run barefoot on a track infield, a treadmill, or even smooth asphalt—as always, be gradual in building up barefoot time and listen to your body. If something feels unusual or any type of pain develops as you adapt, back off and allow adaptation to occur.

f. **Try a barefoot-style or minimalist shoe.** If the thought of running barefoot is too much for you, slowly building up to a few miles a week in a minimalist shoe is another excellent way to work on your form. The past few years have seen the introduction of a wide variety of minimal shoe models, so plenty of options are available. Some people find that they like running in these shoes so much that they transition to them for the bulk of their miles, others use them more sparingly on just a run or two per week. Find the mix that provides maximum benefit and minimal risk to you.

g. **Find a coach.** A good running coach can help you tune your form—obtaining outside feedback might make form change easier and safer than going it alone.

12. **Get strong and flexible.** Less-than-optimal running form and injuries can often be the result of a muscular imbalance or poor muscle strength in the feet, legs, or hips. Try working on being able to better control balance, increasing foot strength, and getting muscle imbalances under control. On being flexible, this is not a function of stretching before you work out or race, but instead concerns restrictions in flexibility that arise from daily activity. For example, tight hip flexors from sitting all day can negatively impact your running. See a professional for a strength and flexibility screen if you feel it's warranted.

13. **Practice good eating habits.** It's important to remember that one of the best ways to make your running easier is to keep your weight down (but not so low that it becomes unhealthy). Shooting for a PR in your next marathon? It's far more likely that losing a few pounds will get you closer to your goal than shaving a few ounces off your shoes. Eat healthy, natural foods, and make your best attempt to limit your overindulgences and avoid the usual junk-food villains.

So how does one conclude a book on running? We suspect that the best way is to end with the simplest of all messages, and one that can apply to all runners, from the beginner to elite. Running should be enjoyed, not painfully endured. Running is in all of our DNA. So listen to your body, respect its needs, and treat it well. In turn, your body will ensure that running is the gift that keeps on giving.

Sources Cited

CHAPTER 1

Wrangham, R. *Catching Fire: How Cooking Made Us Human.* New York: Basic Books, 2009.

Newton, A. *Running.* London: H. F. & G. Witherby, 1935.

Shea, JJ. 2006. The Origins of Lithic Projectile Point Technology: Evidence from Africa, the Levant, and Europe. *Journal of Archaeological Science* 33(6):823–846.

Carrier, DR. 1984. The Energetic Paradox of Human Running and Hominid Evolution. *Current Anthropology* 25(4):483–495.

Bramble DM, Lieberman DE. 2004. Endurance running and the Evolution of *Homo. Nature* 432:345–352.

Lieberman DE, Bramble DM. 2007. The evolution of marathon running capabilities in humans. *Sports Med* 37:288–90.

Lieberman, DE, Bramble, DM, Raichlen, DA, Shea, JJ. Brains, Brawn, and the Evolution of Human Endurance Running Capabilities. 2009. In: Grine, FE, Fleagle, JG, Leakey, RE (Eds.), *The First Humans—Origin and Early Evolution of the Genus Homo.* Stony Brook, NY. Springer, pp. 77–92.

Pickering TR, Bunn HT. 2007. The endurance running hypothesis and hunting and scavenging in savanna-woodlands. *Journal of Human Evolution* 53(4):434–438.

Bunn HT, Pickering, TR. 2010. Bovid mortality profiles in paleoecological context falsify hypotheses of endurance running–hunting and passive scavenging by early Pleistocene hominins. *Quaternary Research* 74:395–404.

Lieberman DE, Bramble DM, Raichlen DA, Shea JJ. 2007. The evolution of endurance running and the tyranny of ethnography: A reply to Pickering and Bunn. *Journal of Human Evolution* 53:434–437.

Pontzer H, Raichlen DA, Sockol MD. 2009. The metabolic cost of walking in humans, chimpanzees, and early hominins. *Journal of Human Evolution* 56:43–54.

Novacheck TF. 1998. The biomechanics of running. *Gait and Posture* 7:77–95.

Ker RF, Bennett MB, Bibby SR, Kester RC, Alexander RM. 1987. The spring in the arch of the human foot. *Nature* 325:147–149.

Lieberman DE, Raichlen DA, Pontzer H, Bramble DM, Cutright-Smith E. 2006. The human gluteus maximus and its role in running. *The Journal of Experimental Biology* 209:2143–2155.

CHAPTER 2

Chakravarty EF, Hubert HB, Lingala VB, Fries JF. 2008. Reducing Disability and Mortality Among Aging Runners: A 21-Year Longitudinal Study. *Archives of Internal Medicine* 168(15):1638–1646.

van Gent RN, Siem M, van Middelkoop M, van Os AG, Bierma-Zeinstra SMA, Koes BW. 2007. Incidence and determinants of lower extremity running injuries in long distance runners: a systematic review. *British Journal of Sports Medicine* 41:469–480.

Van Mechelen W. 1992. Running injuries. A review of the epidemiological literature. *Sports Medicine* 14:320–35.

Satterthwaite P, Norton R, Larmer P, Robinson E.. 1999. Risk factors for injuries and other health problems sustained in a marathon. *British Journal of Sports Medicine* 33:22–26.

Wen DY, Puffer JC, Schmalzried TP. 1998. Injuries in runners: a prospective study of alignment. *Clinical Journal of Sports Medicine* 8:187–94.

Taunton JE, Ryan MB, Clement DB, McKenzie DC, Lloyd-Smith DR, Zumbo BD. 2003. A prospective study of running injuries: the Vancouver Sun Run "In Training" clinics. *British Journal of Sports Medicine* 37:239–44.

Newton, A. *Running*. London: H. F. & G. Witherby, 1935.

Cavanagh PR. *The Running Shoe Book*. Mountain View, CA: Anderson World, 1980.

Macera C, Pate R, Powell K, Jackson KL, Kendrick JS, Craven TE. 1989. Predicting lower-extremity injuries among habitual runners. *Archives of Internal Medicine* 149:2565–2568.

Walter SD, Hart LE, McIntosh JM, Sutton MB. 1989. The Ontario cohort study of running-related injuries. *Archives of Internal Medicine* 149:2561–2564.

Chakravarty EF, Hubert HB, Lingala VB, Zatarain E, Fries JF. 2008. Long Distance Running and Knee Osteoarthritis A Prospective Study. *American Journal of Preventative Medicine* 35(2):133–138.

Noehren B, Davis I, Hamill J. 2007. Prospective study of the biomechanical factors associated with iliotibial band syndrome. *Clinical Biomechanics* 22:951–956.

Buist I, Bredeweg, Bessem B, van Mechelen W, Lemmink KAPM, Diercks RL. 2010. Incidence and risk factors of running-related injuries during preparation for a 4-mile recreational running event. *British Journal of Sports Medicine* 44:598–604.

Hreljac A. 2004. Impact and Overuse Injuries in Runners. *Medicine and Science in Sport and Exercise* 36(5):845–849.

CHAPTER 3

Higdon H. *Smart Running: Expert Advice On Training, Motivation, Injury Prevention, Nutrition, and Good Health.* Emmaus, Pennsylvania: Rodale Books, 1998.

Crowell HP, Milner CE, Hamill J, Davis IS. 2010. Reducing Impact Loading During Running With the Use of Real-Time Visual Feedback. *Journal of Orthopaedic & Sports Physical Therapy* 40(4):206–213.

Crowell HP, Davis IS. 2011. Gait retraining to reduce lower extremity loading in runners. *Clinical Biomechanics* 26:78–83.

Heiderscheit B. 2011. Gait Retraining for Runners: In Search of the Ideal. *Journal of Orthopaedic & Sports Physical Therapy* 41(12):909–910.

Lieberman D E, Venkadesan M, Werbel WA, Daoud AI, D'Andrea S, Davis, IS, Ojiambo Mang'Eni R, Pitsiladis Y. 2010. Foot strike patterns and collision forces in habitually barefoot versus shod runners. *Nature* 463:531–535.

D'Aout K, Pataky TC, De Clerq D, Aerts P. 2009. The effects of habitual footwear use: foot shape and function in native barefoot walkers. *Footwear Science* 1(2):81–94.

Mays SA. 2005. Paleopathological study of hallux valgus. *American Journal of Physical Anthropology* 126:139–149.

Mafart B. 2007. Hallux valgus in a historical French population: Paleopathological study of 605 first metatarsal bones. *Joint Bone Spine* 74:166–170.

Leno JB. *The Art of Boot and Shoemaking, A Practical Handbook.* London: Crosby Lockwood and Co., 1885.

Munson EL. *The Soldier's Foot and the Military Shoe.* Wisconsin: The George Santa Publishing Company, 1912.

Csapo R, Maganaris CN, Seynnes OR, Narici MV. 2010. On muscle, tendon, and high heels. *Journal of Experimental Biology* 213:2582–2588.

Franz JR, Dicharry J, Jackson K, Wilder RP, Kerrigan DC. 2008. The Influence of Arch Supports on Knee Torques Relevant to Knee Osteoarthritis. *Medicine & Science in Sport & Exercise* 40(5):913–917.

Kerrigan DC, Franz JR, Keenan GS, Dicharry J, Della Croce U, Wilder RP. 2009. The Effect of Running Shoes on Lower Extremity Joint Torques. *PM&R* 1:1058–1063.

Newton, A. *Running*. London: H. F. & G. Witherby, 1935.

Ferris DP, Louie M, Farley CT. 1998. Running in the real world: adjusting leg stiffness for different surfaces. *Proceedings of the Royal Society of London* B 265:989–994.

Ferris DP, Liang K, Farley CT. 1999. Runners adjust leg stiffness for their first step on a new running surface. *Journal of Biomechanics* 32:787–794.

Nigg BM. *Biomechanics of Sports Shoes*. Calgary: Topline Printing Inc., 2010.

Nigg BM, Wakeling JM. Impact Forces and Muscle Tuning: A New Paradigm. *Exercise and Sport Sciences Reviews* 29(1):37–41.

Dixon SJ, Collop AC, Batt ME. 2000. Surface effects on ground reaction forces and lower extremity kinematics in running. *Medicine & Science in Sports & Exercise* 32(11):1919–1926.

Feehery RV. 1986. The Biomechanics of Running on Different Surfaces. *Clinics in Podiatric Medicine and Surgery* 3(4):649–659.

Walter SD, Hart LE, McIntosh JM, Sutton JR. 1989. The Ontario Cohort Study of Running-Related Injuries. *Archives of Internal Medicine* 149:2561–2564.

Macera CA, Pate RR, Powell KE, Jackson KL, Kendrick JS, Craven TE. 1989. Predicting Lower-Extremity Injuries Among Habitual Runners. *Archives of Internal Medicine* 149:2565–2568.

Bascomb N. *The Perfect Mile: Three Athletes, One Goal, and Less Than Four Minutes to Achieve It*. New York: Houghton Mifflin Company, 2004.

CHAPTER 4

Strasser, J.B and Beckland, L. *Swoosh: Unauthorized Story of Nike and the Men Who Played There*. Harper Business, 1993.

Moore, Kenny. Bowerman and the Men of Oregon: *The Story of Oregon's Legendary Coach and Nike's Cofounder*. Rodale Books, 2007.

Bilger, Burkhard, "Sole Survivor." *New Yorker*, February 14, 2005

Stewart. Steele, M.D. Footgear—Its History, Uses and Abuses. *Clinical Ortho-paedics and Related Research*, October 1972:119–130

Leno JB. *The Art of Boot and Shoemaking, A Practical Handbook*. London: Crosby Lockwood and Co., 1885.

Kastner, Charles. *Bunion Derby: The 1928 Footrace Across America*. University of New Mexico Press, 2007.

Cavanagh PR. *The Running Shoe Book*. Mountain View, CA: Anderson World, 1980.

Smit, Barbara. *Sneaker Wars: The Enemy Brothers Who Founded Adidas and Puma and the Family Feud That Forever Changed the Business of Sports*. Harper Perennial, 2009.

Gilbert, Matthew Sakiestewa. "Hopi Footraces and American Marathons, 1912–1930." *American Quarterly* (March 2010), Vol. 62, No. 1:77–101.

Nabokov, Peter. *Indian Running: Native American History and Tradition* Ancient City Pr, 1987.

CHAPTER 5

Galloway, Jeff. *Galloway's Book on Running* Shelter Publications; 2nd edition, 2002.

Strasser, J.B and Beckland, L. *Swoosh: Unauthorized Story of Nike and the Men Who Played There*. Harper Business, 1993.

Bowerman WJ, Harris WE. *Jogging*. New York: Grosset & Dunlap, 1967.

Cavanagh PR. *The Running Shoe Book*. Mountain View, CA: Anderson World, 1980.

CHAPTER 6

Ryan MB, Valiant GA, McDonald K, Taunton JE. 2011. The effect of three different levels of footwear stability on pain outcomes in women runners: a randomised control trial. *British Journal of Sports Medicine* 45(9):715–721.

Knapik JJ, Swedler DI, Grier TL, Hauret KG, Bullock SH, Williams KW, Darakjy SS, Lester ME, Tobler SK, Jones BH. 2009. Injury reduction effectiveness of selecting running shoes based on plantar shape. *Journal of Strength and Conditioning Research* 23:685–697.

Knapik JJ, Trone DW, Swedler DI, Villasenor A, Bullock SH, Schmied E, Bockelman T, Han P, Jones BH. 2010. Injury reduction effectiveness of assigning running shoes based on plantar shape in Marine Corps basic training. *The American Journal of Sports Medicine* 38:1759–1767.

Knapik JJ, Brosch LC, Venuto M, Swedler DI Bullock SH, Gaines LS, Murphy RJ, Tchandja J, Jones BH. 2010. Effect on Injuries of Assigning Shoes Based on Foot Shape in Air Force Basic Training. *American Journal of Preventative Medicine* 38:S197–S211.

Cowan DN, Jones BH, Robinson JR. 1993. Foot morphologic characteristics and risk of exercise-related injury. *Archives of Family Medicine* 2:773–777.

Williams DS, McClay IS, Hamill J. 2001. Arch structure and injury patterns in runners. *Clinical Biomechanics* 16:341–347.

Nigg BM, Cole GK, Nachbauer W. 1993. Effects of arch height of the foot on angular motion of the lower extremities in running. *Journal of Biomechanics* 26:909–916.

Dicharry JM, Franz, JR, Della Croce U, Wilder RP, Riley PO, Kerrigan DC. 2009. Differences in Static and Dynamic Measures in Evaluation of Talonavicular Mobility in Gait. *Journal of Orthopaedic and Sports Physical Therapy* 39(8):628–634.

Stacoff A, Nigg BM, Reinschmidt C, van den Bogert AJ, Lundberg A. 2000. Tibiocalcaneal kinematics of barefoot versus shod running. *Journal of Biomechanics* 33:1387–1395.

James SL, Bates BT, Osternig LR. 1978. Injuries to runners. *American Journal of Sports Medicine* 6:40–49.

Wen DY, Puffer JC, Schmalzried TP. 1998. Injuries in Runners: A Prospective Study of Alignment. *Clinical Journal of Sports Medicine* 8(3):187–194.

Nigg BM. 2001. The Role of Impact Forces and Foot Pronation: A New Paradigm. *Clinical Journal of Sports Medicine* 11:2–9.

Lun V, Meeuwisee WH, Stergiou P, Stefanyshyn D. 2004. Relation between running injury and static lower limb alignment in recreational runners. *British Journal of Sports Medicine* 38:576–580.

Hreljac A, Marshall RN, Hume PA. 2000. Evaluation of lower extremity overuse injury potential in runners. *Medicine & Science in Sport & Exercise* 32(9):1635–1641.

Viitasalo JT, Kvist M. 1983. Some biomechanical aspects of the foot and ankle in athletes with and without shin splints. *American Journal of Sports Medicine* 11(3):125–30.

Hinterman B, Nigg BM. 1998. Pronation in Runners: Implications for Injuries. *Sports Medicine* 26(3):169–176.

Nigg BM. *Biomechanics of Sports Shoes*. Calgary: Topline Printing Inc., 2010.

CHAPTER 7

Fixx JF. *The Complete Book of Running*. New York: Random House, 1977.

Osler T. *Serious Runners Handbook*. Mountain View, California: World Publications, Inc., 1978.

Dreyer D, Dreyer K. *Chi Running*. New York: Simon & Schuster, 2009.

Henderson J. *Running 101*. Champaign, Illinois: Human Kinetics, 2000.

Pirie G. *Running Fast and Injury Free*. United Kingdom: JS Gilbody, 2002.

Bowerman WJ, Harris WE. *Jogging*. New York: Grosset & Dunlap, 1967.

Kerr BA, Beauchamp L, Fisher V, Neil R. 1983. Footstrike patterns in distance running. In: Kerr BA (Ed.), *Biomechanical Aspects of Sport Shoes and Playing Surfaces: Proceedings of the International Symposium on Biomechanical Aspects of Sport Shoes and Playing Surfaces*. Calgary, Alberta: University Press, pp. 135–142.

Hasegawa H, Yamauchi T, Kraemer WJ. 2007. Foot strike patterns of runners at the 15-Km point during an elite-level half marathon. *Journal of Strength and Conditioning Research* 21:888–893.

Larson PM, Higgins E, Kaminski J, Decker T, Preble J, Lyons D, McIntyre K, Normile A. 2011. Foot strike patterns of recreational and sub-elite runners in a long-distance road race. *Journal of Sports Sciences* 29(15):1665–1673.

Nett T. 1964. Foot plant in running. *Track Technique* 15: 462–463.

Cavanagh PR, Lafortune MA. 1980. Ground reaction forces in distance running. *Journal of Biomechanics* 13:397–406.

Lieberman D E, Venkadesan M, Werbel WA, Daoud AI, D'Andrea S, Davis, IS, Ojiambo Mang'Eni R, Pitsiladis Y. 2010. Foot strike patterns and collision forces in habitually barefoot versus shod runners. *Nature* 463:531–535.

Wegener C, Hunt AE, Vanwanseele B, Burns J, Smith RM. Effect of children's shoes on gait: a systematic review and meta-analysis. *Journal of Foot and Ankle Research* 4:3.

Squadrone R, Gallozzi C. 2009. Biomechanical and physiological comparison of barefoot and two shod conditions in experienced barefoot runners. *Journal of Sports Medicine and Physical Fitness* 49:6–13.

McCarthy C, Porcari JP, Kernoek T, Willson J, Foster C, Anders M. Like Barefoot, Only Better? *ACE Certified News*, September 2011.

Zadpoor AA, Nikooyan AA. 2011. The relationship between lower-extremity stress fractures and the ground reaction force: A systematic review. *Clinical Biomechanics* 26:23–28.

Pohl MB, Hamill J, Davis IS. 2009. Biomechanical and anatomic factors associated with a history of plantar fasciitis in female runners. *Clinical Journal of Sports Medicine* 19:372–376.

Daoud AI, Geissler GJ, Wang F, Saretsky J, Daoud YA, Lieberman DE. 2012. Foot Strike and Injury Rates in Endurance Runners: a retrospective study. *Medicine & Science in Sport & Exercise.* Epub ahead of print.

Nigg BM. *Biomechanics of Sports Shoes.* Calgary: Topline Printing Inc., 2010.

CHAPTER 8

Bishop M, Fiolkowski P, Conrad B, Brunt D, Horodyski M. 2006. Athletic Footwear, Leg Stiffness, and Running Kinematics. *Journal of Athletic Training* 41(4):387–392.

De Wit, B., De Clercq, D. & Aerts, P. (2000). Biomechanical analysis of the stance phase during barefoot and shod running. *Journal of Biomechanics* 33:269–278.

Divert, C., Mornieux, G., Baur, H., Mayer, F. & Belli, A. (2005). Mechanical comparison of barefoot and shod running. *International Journal of Sports Medicine* 26:593–598.

Kerrigan DC, Franz JR, Keenan GS, Dicharry J, Della Croce U, Wilder RP. 2009. The Effect of Running Shoes on Lower Extremity Joint Torques. *PM&R* 1:1058–1063.

Lieberman D E, Venkadesan M, Werbel WA, Daoud AI, D'Andrea S, Davis, IS, Ojiambo Mang'Eni R, Pitsiladis Y. 2010. Foot strike patterns and collision forces in habitually barefoot versus shod runners. *Nature* 463:531–535.

Squadrone R, Gallozzi C. 2009. Biomechanical and physiological comparison of barefoot and two shod conditions in experienced barefoot runners. *Journal of Sports Medicine and Physical Fitness* 49:6–13.

Stacoff A, Nigg BM, Reinschmidt C, van den Bogert AJ, Lundberg A. 2000. Tibiocalcaneal kinematics of barefoot versus shod running. *Journal of Biomechanics* 33(11):1387–1395.

Shrubb AA. *Running and Cross-Country Running.* London: Health and Strength, Ltd., 1908.

Newton, A. *Running.* London: H. F. & G. Witherby, 1935.

Wilt F. *Run Run Run.* Los Altos, CA: Track and Field News, 1964.

Bowerman WJ, Harris WE. *Jogging.* New York: Grosset & Dunlap, 1967.

Sheehan GA. *Dr. George Sheehan's Medical Advice for Runners.* Mountain View, CA: World Publications, 1978.

Cavanagh PR. *The Running Shoe Book*. Mountain View, CA: Anderson World, 1980.

Robbins SE, Gouw GJ. 1990. Athletic Footwear and Chronic Overloading: A Brief Review. *Sports Medicine* 9(2):76–85.

von Tscharner V, Goepfert B, Nigg BM. 2003. Changes in EMG signals for the muscle tibialis anterior while running barefoot or with shoes resolved by non-linearly scaled wavelets. *Journal of Biomechanics* 36:1169–1176.

Derrick TR, Hamill J, Caldwell GE. 1998. Energy absorption of impacts during running at various stride lengths. *Medicine & Science in Sport & Exercise* 30(1):128–135.

Hamill J, Derrick TR, Holt KG. 1995. Shock attenuation and stride frequency during running. *Human Movement Science* 14:45–60.

Hamill J, Bates BT, Knutzen KM, Sawhill JA. 1983. Variations in ground reaction force parameters at different running speeds. *Human Movement Science* 2:47–56.

Munro CF, Miller DI, Fuglevand AJ. 1987. Ground reaction forces in running: A reexamination. *Journal of Biomechanics* 20(2):147–155.

Clarke TE, Cooper LB, Hamill CL, Clark DE. The effect of varied stride rate upon shank deceleration in running. *Journal of Sports Sciences* 3:41–49.

Heiderscheit BC, Chumanov ES, Michalski MP, Wille CM, Ryan MB. 2011. Effects of Step Rate Manipulation on Joint Mechanics during Running. *Medicine & Science in Sports & Exercise* 43:296–302.

Edwards WB, Taylor D, Rudolph TJ, Gillette JC, Derrick TR. 2009. Effects of stride Length and Running Mileage on a Probabilistic Stress Fracture Model. *Medicine & Science in Sports & Exercise* 41(12):2177–2184.

Jerome J. *The Sweet Spot in Time: The Search for Athletic Perfection*. New York: Breakaway Books, 1980.

Daniels J. *Daniels' Running Formula*. Champaign, IL: Human Kinetics, 2005.

Cavanagh PR, Williams KR. The effect of stride length variation on oxygen uptake during distance running. *Medicine & Science in Sports & Exercise* 14(1):30–35.

Cavanagh PR, Kram R. 1989. Stride length in distance running: velocity, body dimensions, and added mass effects. *Medicine & Science in Sports & Exercise* 21(4):467–479.

Van Mechelen W. 1992. Running injuries. A review of the epidemiological literature. *Sports Medicine* 14:320–35.

Morgan D, Martin P, Craib M, Caruso C, Clifton R, Hopewell R. 1994. Effect of step length optimization on the aerobic demand of running. *Journal of Applied Physiology* 77(1):245–251.

Crowell HP, Milner CE, Hamill J, Davis IS. 2010. Reducing Impact Loading During Running With the Use of Real-Time Visual Feedback. *Journal of Orthopaedic & Sports Physical Therapy* 40(4):206–213.

Crowell HP, Davis IS. 2011. Gait retraining to reduce lower extremity loading in runners. *Clinical Biomechanics* 26:78–83.

Franz JR, Paylo KW, Dicharry J, Riley PO, Kerrigan DC. Changes in the coordination of hip and pelvis kinematics with mode of locomotion. *Gait & Posture* 29:494–498.

CHAPTER 9

Wrangham, R. *Catching Fire: How Cooking Made Us Human.* New York: Basic Books, 2009.

Mozaffarian D, Tao Hao PH, Rimm EB, Willett WC, Hu FB. 2011. Changes in diet and lifestyle and long-term weight gain in women and men. *New England Journal of Medicine* 364:2392–2404.

O'Keefe JH, Vogel R, Lavie CJ, Cordain L. 2010. Achieving Hunter-gatherer Fitness in the 21st Century: Back to the Future. *The American Journal of Medicine* 123(12):1082–1086.

Noakes T. 2003. *Lore of Running,* 4th ed, Champaign, Illinois: Human Kinetics.

Teunissen LPJ, Grabowski A, Kram R. 2007. Effects of independently altering body weight and body mass on the metabolic cost of running. *Journal of Experimental Biology* 210:4418–4427.

McDougall, Christopher. *Born to Run: A Hidden Tribe, Superathletes, and the Greatest Race the World Has Never Seen.* Knopf, 2009.

Maffetone, Phil. *The Big Book of Health and Fitness.* Skyhorse Publishing, 2011.

Pollan, Michael. *In Defense of Food: An Eater's Manifesto.* Penguin, 2009.

Acknowledgments

We are indebted to the many people who made this book possible. Special thanks go to Daniel Lieberman and Jay Dicharry, both of whom graciously took the time to answer our many questions on the topics of human evolution, running injuries, and running form. Deep kudos must be given to Dr. Mark Cucuzzella, who contributed written material on shoe fitting, and who was a constant source of support and advice on running form. If only we could all run like him. "Dr. Mark," as many runners who have attended his form clinics prefer to call him, has perfected natural running after years of trial and error. He's an inspiration to anyone who wants to improve as a runner.

Pete would like to thank Amby Burfoot, Brett Coapland, Blaise Dubois, Alex Hutchinson, Casey Kerrigan, Steve Magness, Christopher McDougall, and the crew from the BFT forum for always interesting and thoughtful discussions on running form, injuries, and footwear. Also, special thanks to the readers of Runblogger.com for serving as a sounding board for much of what is written here—your comments and thoughts are always appreciated! Special thanks to my coauthor Bill Katovsky for offering me the opportunity to write this book—it would not have happened without him. Bill, you did a great job reining me in when I attempted to get too technical, and your help and advice along the way has been invaluable. If this book is readable, it's because of you! Finally, and most of all, a huge thanks to my wife, Erin, and children—Anders, Emma, and Ben—for putting up with dad's endless droning about running shoes, and for supporting him through what at times has been a long and arduous process.

Bill's turn: Interesting how life states its unpredictable case. Three years ago, I wasn't running. Now it's all I want to think about, and the way I got to this good place was by immersing myself in this world of like-minded individuals, who are equally determined to figure things out on their own. I met Pete online via *Runblogger*. I had just started my own blog, Zero-Drop.com, and I immediately knew that it was only a matter of time before the running community would acknowledge him as an authoritative expert when it came to matters of form and footwear. As a part-time literary agent, I pitched the idea to Pete that he should write a book on running, but in the end, we decided to collaborate as co-authors. It was a smart decision. I learned a lot from him as *Tread Lightly* gradually took shape. He brought much-needed scientific rigor to a topic that too often has been sidetracked by opinion and conjecture.

Others who have assisted me along the way: Dr. Phil Maffetone, who is wise, thoughtful, and usually right; Dave Low, for his encouragement; Nick Pang, my colleague at the Natural Running Center and founder of the website Minimalist Running Shoes; Dr. Steve Gangemi, a.k.a. Sock Doc, who often gets it, and all I can say is that injury-prone runners just might want to heed his non-conventional counsel. Finally, *Tread Lightly* required a publisher to believe in the concept. So thank you, Tony Lyons of Skyhorse Publishing.

Index